medical
examination review — volume 11

Pediatrics
FIFTH EDITION

1060 Multiple Choice Questions
with Referenced Explanatory Answers

By
Hershel P. Wall, M.D., F.A.A.P.
Professor of Pediatrics
Director, Ambulatory Pediatric Service

Marvin I. Gottlieb, M.D., Ph.D., F.A.A.P.
Professor of Pediatrics
Chief, Section of Developmental and
Behavioral Pediatrics

Carole M. Perry, M.D., F.A.A.P.
Formerly, Assistant Professor of Pediatrics
The University of Tennessee Center for the
Health Sciences/ Le Bonheur Children's Hospital
Memphis, Tennessee

 Medical Examination Publishing Co., Inc.
an Excerpta Medica company

GARDEN CITY, NEW YORK

/

notice

The editor(s) and/or author(s) and the publisher of this book have made
every effort to ensure that all therapeutic modalities that are recommended are in accordance with accepted standards at the time of pub-
lication.

The drugs specified within this book may not have specific approval by
the Food and Drug Administration in regard to the indications and dos-
ages that are recommended by the editor(s) and/or author(s). The manu-
facturer's package insert is the best source of current prescribing information.

Preface

This fifth edition of *Medical Examination Review, Volume 11, Pediatrics* has been substantially revised and updated to keep in step with current trends in medical education and the continuing expansion of scientific knowledge. It is designed to help you prepare for course examinations, National Boards Part II, the Federation Licensing Examination (FLEX), the Educational Commission on Foreign Medical Graduates examination (ECFMG), the Visa Qualifying Examination (VQE), and other objective exams.

The range of subjects included in this volume is based on the content outline of the National Board of Medical Examiners, which develops the question pool for the tests mentioned above, and reflects the scope and depth of what is taught in medical schools today. The questions themselves are organized in broad categories, to give you a representative sampling of the material covered in course work, while helping you define those general areas to which you need to devote attention. For your convenience in selective study, the answers (with commentary and references) follow each section of questions.

Each question has been scrutinized by specialists to verify that it is relevant and current. The authors' care in item construction gives you questions that will provide good practice in familiarizing yourself with the format of objective-type tests. Questions of each type — one best response, matching, multiple true-false, and so on — are grouped together. They are modelled as closely as possible after those used by the Board.

Using this book, you may identify areas of strength and weakness in your own command of the subject. Specific references to widely-used textbooks allow you to return to the authoritative source for further study. This volume supplements the lettered answers with brief explanations intended to prompt you to think about the choices — correct and incorrect, to put the answers in broadened perspective, and to add to your fund of knowledge. A complete bibliography appears at the end of the book. The questions and answers, taken together, emphasize problem solving and application of underlying principles as well as retention of factual knowledge.

Contents

disclaimer

The authors have made every effort to thoroughly verify the answers to the questions which appear on the following pages. However, as in any text, some inaccuracies and ambiguities may occur; therefore, if in doubt, please consult your references.

The Publisher

I: Perinatology

DIRECTIONS: Each of the questions or incomplete statements below is followed by five suggested answers or completions. Select the **one** that is **BEST** in each case.

1. The hormone that promotes utilization of fat stores as fuel and increases the material capacity for sparing protein and glucose is
    A. chorionic gonadotrophin
    B. progesterone
    . C. placental lactogen
    D. estrogen
    E. testosterone

2. At birth, the blood volume is approximately
    A. 65 ml/kg body weight
    . B. 85 ml/kg body weight
    C. 110 ml/kg body weight
    D. 125 ml/kg body weight
    E. 150 ml/kg body weight

3. The neonate is relatively resistant to ketosis during periods of caloric deprivation. The best explanation for this is
    A. greater glycogen stores in muscle
    . B. fat depot comprises a greater percentage of total body weight in the neonate than in the older child
    C. lack of fat-mobilizing enzymes
    D. more saturated character of neonatal fat
    E. a lower metabolic rate

4. Which of the following signs is pathognomonic of entero-colitis?
   A. Pneumoperitoneum
   ·B. Bloody stools and abdominal distension
   C. Bile-stained vomitus
   D. Pneumatosis cystoides intestinalis
   E. Ileal perforation

5. All of the following may be sources of blood in the vomitus of a two-day-old newborn EXCEPT
   A. placental blood swallowed at delivery
   B. suctioning
   C. breast feeding
   ~D. irritation caused by silver nitrate
   E. gastrointestinal hemorrhage

6. The Apt test is used for what purpose?
   A. Crude test for carbon monoxide poisoning
   B. Semi-quantitative test for lead poisoning
   ꞋC. Qualitative test for fetal hemoglobin
   D. Screening test for S hemoglobin
   E. Test for blood viscosity

7. Therapy for neonatal necrotizing enterocolitis may include all of the following EXCEPT
   ~A. systemic antibodies
   B. surgical resection
   C. discontinuance of oral feeding
   D. correction of low blood volume
   E. use of elemental enteral feedings

8. In most series of patients with necrotizing enterocolitis, the mortality is
   ꞌ A. 10%
   B. 20%
   C. 30%
   D. in excess of 50%
   E. 100%

9. Meconium ileus in the newborn is best treated by
   A. enzyme replacement
   B. barium enema
   C. surgery
   D. irrigation of gut with N-acetylcysteine
   E. phosphate enema

10. In neonates, icterus of the sclera or skin is usually NOT apparent until serum bilirubin exceeds
    A. 2 mg/dl
    B. 5 mg/dl
    C. 8 mg/dl
    D. 10 mg/dl
    E. 15 mg/dl

11. What percentage of excreted bilirubin results from breakdown of mature circulating erythrocytes?
    A. 95%
    B. 70%
    C. 99%
    D. 80%
    E. 50%

12. All of the following statements are true concerning serum transport of bilirubin EXCEPT
    A. it is transported primarily bound to albumin
    B. sulfonamides compete for binding sites
    C. one mole of albumin can bind approximately 1 mole of bilirubin in vivo
    D. multiple binding sites exist
    E. the first binding site has greatest affinity

13. All of the following statements are true concerning urobilinogen metabolism EXCEPT
    A. it is a result of bilirubin in the lumen of the distal small intestine
    B. end products of its metabolism are urobilin and stercobilin
    C. amounts in urine may be increased in severe hepatitis
    D. amounts in urine may be increased in biliary atresia
    E. bacteria are involved in its production

14. All of the following are characteristic of the digestive system of a newborn EXCEPT
    A. fat and large milk curds delay emptying time of stomach
    B. by 12 hours after birth, air can be found in the small intestine
    C. absorption of protein is poor until several weeks after birth
    D. hydrochloric acid is present in adequate amounts in the neonate
    E. starch may not be completely digested

15. Craniotabes may be present in all of the following EXCEPT
    A. premature infants
    B. rickets
    C. hydrocephalus
    D. normal infants
    E. the neonate showing symptoms of syphilis

16. Hypertrophy and hyperplasia of the islets of Langerhans have been found in infants of mothers with diabetes and in infants with which of the following conditions?
    A. Erythroblastosis fetalis
    B. Congenital rubella
    C. Congenital toxoplasmosis
    D. Cytomegalovirus infection
    E. Herpes simplex infection

17. All of the following drugs administered during pregnancy have been associated with masculinization of the female fetus, EXCEPT
    A. methyltestosterone
    B. progesterone
    C. stilbestrol
    D. propylthiouracil
    E. 17-alpha-ethinyl-19-nortestosterone

18. The chemical analysis of choice to determine fetal maturity in amniotic fluid is
    A. creatinine and lecithin
    B. bilirubin
    C. urea
    D. DNA and amino acids
    E. total lipids

19. Polyhydramnios is frequently associated with fetal malformations, including
    A. renal agenesis
    B. anencephaly
    C. pulmonary hypoplasia
    D. urethral atresia
    E. amnion nodosum

20. Mongolian spots are characterized by all of the following, EXCEPT
    A. permanence
    B. they are usually of a slate-blue pigmentation
    C. they are generally observed over the buttocks
    D. the area of pigmentation is well demarcated
    E. they are not associated with trisomy syndromes

21. Localized edema in a newborn is suggestive of all of the following EXCEPT
    A. prematurity
    B. hydrops fetalis
    C. congenital nephrosis
    D. congenital malformation of the lymphatic system
    E. fluid overload

22. Epstein's pearls on the hard palate of a newborn should be treated with
    A. topical antibiotics
    B. topical steroids
    C. excision and drainage
    D. no therapy
    E. hydrogen peroxide

23. The newborn's eyes can be protected by the instillation of what percentage of silver nitrate drops?
    A. 1%
    B. 3%
    C. 5%
    D. 10%
    E. 20%

24. In the United States, the incidence of twins is approximately
   A. one of 50 pregnancies
   B. one of 85 pregnancies
   C. one of 115 pregnancies
   D. one of 200 pregnancies
   E. one of 300 pregnancies

25. Which of the following countries has the highest birth rate of infants weighing less than 2500 grams?
   A. Netherlands
   B. Denmark
   C. Norway
   D. United States (white)
   E. Sweden

26. All of the following physical signs may be useful in estimating gestational age at birth EXCEPT
   A. there are only one or two transverse skin creases on the sole of the foot until 36 weeks of gestation
   B. the breast nodule is usually not palpable at 33 or 34 weeks
   C. the breast nodule is usually 4 to 10 mm in term infants
   D. the testes are descending and rugae cover the entire scrotal surface by 34 weeks
   E. texture of the scalp hair

27. Postterm infants are defined as having a
   A. birthweight of 3,600 gm
   B. birthweight of 4,000 gm
   C. gestational age of 41 weeks
   D. birthweight more than 4,500 gm
   E. gestational age more than 42 weeks

28. Postterm postmature infants are characterized by all of the following EXCEPT
   A. lanugo
   B. long nails
   C. abundant scalp hair
   D. increased alertness
   E. loss of subcutaneous tissue

29. Caput succedaneum is characterized by all of the following EXCEPT
- **A.** a diffuse, edematous swelling of the soft tissues of the scalp, involving the portion presenting during vertex delivery
- **B.** it may extend across midline
- **C.** it may extend across suture lines
- **D.** edema usually disappears within two to three months
- **E.** the scalp overlying the area may show mild bruising

30. Neonatal intracranial hemorrhage is more frequently found in all of the following EXCEPT
- **A.** premature infants
- **B.** infants born by cesarean section
- **C.** infants with cephalic presentation
- **D.** infants delivered by mechanical aids other than low forceps
- **E.** infants experiencing asphyxia

31. In Duchenne-Erb paralysis, the injury is limited to
- **A.** first and second cervical nerves
- **B.** third and fourth cervical nerves
- **C.** fifth and sixth cervical nerves
- **D.** first and second thoracic nerves
- **E.** first through fourth cervical nerves

32. Fetal narcosis may result from administration of large doses of certain drugs to the mother shortly before delivery. All of the following may produce narcosis EXCEPT
- **A.** barbiturates
- **B.** Demerol
- **C.** tranquilizers
- **D.** Pitocin
- **E.** general anesthetics

33. Idiopathic respiratory distress syndrome is usually NOT associated with
- **A.** full-term infants
- **B.** infants of diabetic mothers (delivered before 37 weeks)
- **C.** antepartum vaginal bleeding
- **D.** infants weighing less than 2,500 grams
- **E.** infants born before 37 weeks gestation

34. A newborn exhibits respiratory distress, distention of neck veins, low blood pressure, hyperresonance, and diminished breath sounds over one side of the chest, and subcutaneous emphysema. The most likely diagnosis is
    A. hyaline membrane disease
    B. staphylococcal pneumonia
    C. pneumothorax and pneumomediastinum
    D. primary atelectasis
    E. diaphragmatic hernia

35. Massive pulmonary hemorrhage has been associated with all of the following EXCEPT
    A. hyaline membrane disease
    B. kernicterus
    C. cold injury
    D. massive meconium aspiration
    E. breech delivery

36. In a newborn with oral moniliasis, the most common primary source of infection is
    A. maternal source (vaginal)
    B. contaminated fomites
    C. following use of $AgNo_3$
    D. contact by hospital carriers
    E. systemic antibiotic therapy

37. Meconium impaction is associated with
    A. cretinism
    B. cystic fibrosis
    C. thrush
    D. hyaline membrane disease
    E. trisomy 21 syndrome

38. Persistent jaundice during the first month of life may be associated with all of the following EXCEPT
    A. cytomegalic inclusion disease
    B. congenital atresia of the bile ducts
    C. galactosemia
    D. Rh incompatibility
    E. penicillin treatment

39. All of the following are characteristic of jaundice associated with breast feeding EXCEPT
    A. significant elevations of unconjugated bilirubin
    B. a rapid fall in serum bilirubin after discontinuation of nursing
    C. nursing can be resumed after several days without return of hyperbilirubinemia
    D. significant elevations of conjugated bilirubin
    E. kernicterus has never been reported to occur as a result of breast-milk jaundice alone

40. In term infants, the clinical manifestations of kernicterus usually appear within
    A. two to five days
    B. fourteen to 21 days
    C. three to five months
    D. six to eight months
    E. one to two years

41. "Bronze Baby syndrome" is associated with
    A. infants undergoing phototherapy for hyperbilirubinemia
    B. excessive use of Chloromycetin in an infant
    C. excessive use of vitamin A during infancy
    D. use of iodine in cauterizing umbilical cord
    E. urinary track infection in the neonate

42. Among first pregnancies, which of the following percentages approximates the occurrence of hemolytic disease due to Rh incompatibility?
    A. 43%
    B. 35%
    C. 25%
    D. 15%
    E. It rarely occurs

43. During the newborn period, jaundice may result from maternal use of
    A. adrenal corticosteroids
    B. reserpine
    C. sulfisoxazole
    D. LSD
    E. aspirin

44. All of the following are characteristic of a single umbilical artery EXCEPT
   A. presence in about five of 1,000 births
   B. about one-third of such infants have congenital abnormalities
   C. trisomy 21 is frequently found
   D. among twins the rate of occurrence is 35% per 1,000
   E. the associated congenital abnormalities may involve the genitourinary tract

45. Signs and symptoms of neonatal cold injury include all of the following EXCEPT
   A. apathy, refusal of food, and oliguria
   B. immobility, edema, and redness of extremities
   C. facial pallor
   D. hemorrhagic manifestations
   E. scleremic skin changes

46. Withdrawal symptoms in an infant born to an actively addicted mother is usually found
   A. within 24 hours
   B. within 48 hours
   C. on the fifth day
   D. on the seventh day
   E. on the 14th day

47. All of the following are usually associated with cretinism EXCEPT
   A. constipation
   B. prolonged jaundice
   C. lethargy
   D. tetany
   E. hypotonia

48. Hypoglycemia has been observed in newborns
   A. with low birthweights and respiratory distress syndrome
   B. with anoxic injury
   C. with hypothermia
   D. who are small for gestational age
   E. with high PaO_2

DIRECTIONS: For each of the questions or incomplete statements below, **ONE** or **MORE** of the answers or completions given is correct. Select

     A if only *1, 2 and 3* are correct,
     B if only *1 and 3* are correct,
     C if only *2 and 4* are correct,
     D if only *4* is correct,
     E if all are correct.

49. Amniocentesis is useful in establishing the prenatal diagnosis of
    1. Down's syndrome
    2. meningomyelocele
    3. erythroblastosis fetalis
    4. achondroplasia

50. Maternal medications that can cause congenital malformations include
    1. thalidomide
    2. penicillin
    3. amphetamines
    4. insulin

51. Indications for fetal scalp blood sampling for pH, $PaCO_2$ and base excess include
    1. fetal tachycardia
    2. flat baseline on the fetal monitor
    3. late decelerations on the fetal monitor
    4. preeclampsia

52. Fetal malformations that are frequently associated with polyhydramnios include
    1. duodenal atresia
    2. renal atresia
    3. esophageal atresia
    4. pulmonary hypoplasia

53. Factors that are associated with high risk pregnancies are
    1. age of mother less than 16 or more than 40
    2. six previous term pregnancies
    3. maternal diabetes mellitus
    4. malnutrition

Directions Summarized				
A	B	C	D	E
1,2,3	1,3	2,4	4	All are
only	only	only	only	correct

54. Maternal urine estriol determinations can be used to
    1. ascertain gestational age of the fetus
    2. indicate fetal growth retardation
    3. diagnose preeclampsia
    4. serve as an index of placental function

55. Ultrasound can be used during pregnancy to
    1. determine crown rump length
    2. determine fetal sex
    3. determine the biparietal diameter
    4. accurately determine fetal weight

56. Intrauterine fetal growth retardation may be associated with
    1. maternal drug addiction
    2. maternal smoking
    3. fetal viral infection
    4. maternal aspirin abuse

57. Maternal anesthesia and analgesia
    1. never affect the fetus
    2. have been proved to be causes of hyaline membrane disease
    3. are associated with prolonged physiologic jaundice of the newborn
    4. can produce neurologic depression that must be differentiated from anoxic or traumatic birth injury

58. Gestations that produce multiple births
    1. are classified as high risk
    2. are always delivered by cesarean section
    3. can produce infants with discordance in body size at birth
    4. are not associated with the premature onset of labor

I: Perinatology
Answers and Comments

1. C. Placental lactogen, a growth hormone–like substance synthesized by the placenta, is produced by the syncytial trophoblast and enters the maternal circulation. *(REF. 1 — p. 132)*

2. B. At birth, the blood volume is about 85 ml/kg body weight, falling to about 75 ml/kg after the first month. *(REF. 1 — pp. 179–181)*

3. D. Neonates have a greater percentage of saturated fat; this is known to be less readily mobilized than unsaturated fat. During the first year of life unsaturated fat rises rapidly. *(REF. 1 — p. 193)*

4. D. Pneumatosis cystoides intestinalis is considered to be pathognomonic of NEC and is rarely, if ever, associated with other clinical disorders. *(REF. 1 — p. 992)*

5. D. Sources other than the infant's gastrointestinal tract must be sought for in the differential diagnosis of vomited blood in the neonate. Silver nitrate used as G-C prophylaxis is applied directly to the conjunctivae and is not a source of blood in the vomitus. *(REF. 1 — p. 988)*

6. C. The Apt test is useful in distinguishing maternal blood from newborn blood. *(REF. 1 — p. 988)*

7. E. Because of the high mortality associated with necrotizing enterocolitis, aggressive treatment should be initiated. If accompanied by shock, immediate correction is critical to survival. Elemental enteral feeding is contraindicated because of the high osmotic load it imposes on the gut. *(REF. 1 — p. 992)*

8. D. Most series have reported mortality rates exceeding 50%. *(REF. 1 — p. 992)*

9. C. In older children, acetylcysteine irrigators may relieve acute obstructions. Recurrences may be prevented by increasing the dose of pancreatic enzyme supplementation. Neonates tolerate non-surgical treatments poorly. *(REF. 1 — p. 996)*

10. B. Icterus is usually detectable at levels greater than 5 mg/dl. *(REF. 1 — p. 1067)*

11. D. Approximately 80% is derived from normal red blood cell destruction. Heme from muscle contributes approximately 10%. *(REF. 1 — p. 1067)*

12. C. The molar ratio in vivo is 1:2; 1 gram of albumin can bind approximately 16 mg of bilirubin. *(REF. 1 — p. 1068)*

13. D. Amounts in urine decrease or are absent in any condition in which there is obstruction of the flow of bile into the intestinal tract. *(REF. 1 — p. 1073)*

14. C. Absorption of protein is good, as is the absorption of carbohydrates and simple sugars. Fat absorption is decreased until several weeks after birth. *(REF. 2 — pp. 173–187)*

15. D. It is also seen in osteogenesis imperfecta, and craniotabes present near suture lines may be normal. *(REF. 2 — p. 233)*

16. A. Most of the increase appears to be due to an increase in number and size of the beta cells of the islets of Langerhans. The other disorders cited are frequently associated with abortion or premature delivery. *(REF. 2 — p. 380)*

17. D. Propylthiouracil has been associated with fetal goiter and does not cause masculinization of the female fetus. *(REF. 2 — p. 381)*

18. A. Amniotic fluid creatinine and lecithin reflect the maturity of the fetal kidney and lung. After 36 weeks of gestation, the creatinine concentration is at least 1.8 mg/dl of amniotic fluid in 98% of pregnancies, with an anmiotic fluid/maternal plasma creatinine ratio of 3:1 or more. In addition, the lecithin concentration is at least 2 mg/dl, with an amniotic fluid lecithin/sphingomyelin ratio of at least 2.0. *(REF. 2 — p. 382)*

19. B. The polyhydramnios associated with anencephaly may be caused by the faulty formation or excretion of antidiuretic hormone. The other conditions cited are associated with oligohydramnios. *(REF. 2 — pp. 386–387)*

20. A. Mongolian spots usually disappear within the first year of life. There is no increased incidence of these lesions with the various trisomy syndromes. *(REF. 2 — p. 390)*

21. D. Congenital malformations of the lymphatic system are not associated with generalized edema. *(REF. 2 — p. 390)*

22. D. Epstein's pearls are temporary collections of epithelial cells. They are benign and require no therapy. *(REF. 2 — p. 391)*

23. A. The eyes of all infants need to be protected against gonorrheal infection; 1% silver nitrate solution is the best-proved therapy. The other concentrations listed are too strong. *(REF. 2 — p. 395)*

24. B. In the U.S. the incidence of twins is approximately one of 85 pregnancies. *(REF. 2 — p. 401)*

25. D. The United States (white) has the highest incidence at 7.2%. Norway is 5.7%, and the lowest is the Netherlands with a rate of 3.5%. *(REF. 3 — p. 342)*

26. D. The testes are usually not completely descended until after 36 weeks and the scrotal rugae are few and limited to the anterior and inferior aspects of a relatively small scrotum. *(REF. 2 — p. 405)*

27. E. Postterm infants are defined as those born after 42 weeks of gestation, calculated from the mother's last menstrual period. The definition does not depend upon the infant's weight. *(REF. 2 — p. 413)*

28. A. Postterm postmature infants are characterized by an absence of lanugo. *(REF. 2 — p. 413)*

29. D. The edema of caput succedaneum usually disappears within the first few days of life and requires no specific therapy. *(REF. 2 — p. 352)*

30. C. Intracranial hemorrhage is found more often in infants with breech presentation, rather than cephalic presentation. *(REF. 2 — pp. 418–419)*

31. C. In Duchenne-Erb paralysis the injury is limited to the fifth and sixth cervical nerves. The infant loses the power to abduct the arm from the shoulder, to rotate the arm from the shoulder, to rotate the arm externally, and to supinate the forearm. *(REF. 2 — p. 420)*

32. D. All of the agents cited except Pitocin, can cause narcosis. At birth, the infant may be cyanotic, slow to cry and breathe, and have slow respirations. *(REF. 2 — p. 425)*

33. A. Idiopathic respiratory distress syndrome is rare in full-term infants, whereas 10% of all premature infants may have the disease. *(REF. 2 — p. 429)*

34. C. The chest findings suggest a pneumothorax, and subcutaneous emphysema in a newborn most strongly suggests pneumomediastinum. *(REF. 2 — pp. 347–348)*

35. E. Massive pulmonary hemorrhage has been associated with all of the conditions cited except the uncomplicated breech delivery. Bleeding is primarily alveolar and is interstitial in only about one third of the cases. Bleeding may be found in the nose and mouth. *(REF. 2 — p. 440)*

36. A. There is a positive correlation between maternal vaginal and infantile oral moniliasis. This is the primary means of infection in a newborn. *(REF. 2 — p. 441)*

37. B. Meconium ileus is associated with cystic fibrosis. Deficiency of pancreatic enzyme limits normal digestive activities in the intestine. As a result meconium is left in a viscid mucilaginous state, and it clings to the walls of the intestine. Movement is very difficult or impossible. *(REF. 2 — p. 441)*

38. E. All but penicillin therapy have been associated with persistent jaundice during the first month of life, suggesting a disorder called "inspissated bile syndrome". *(REF. 2 — p. 444)*

39. D. Direct bilirubin is not elevated. There is some evidence to suggest that maternal hormonal substances in milk interfere with bilirubin metabolism, but this defect does not involve the excretion of the conjugated form of bilirubin. *(REF. 2 — p. 446)*

40. A. Signs and symptoms of kernicterus usually appear within two to five days after birth in term infants. However, hyperbilirubinemia may cause this syndrome at any time during the neonatal period. *(REF. 2 — p. 446)*

41. A. "Bronze Baby syndrome" refers to a discoloration (dark, grayish-brown) of the skin in infants undergoing phototherapy. Almost all infants exhibiting this discoloration have had a mixed type of hyperbilirubinemia, which is characterized by a significant elevation of direct-reacting bilirubin in the serum and often with evidence of obstructive liver disease. *(REF. 2 — p. 449)*

42. E. Hemolytic disease is rare during a first pregnancy because transfusions of Rh-positive fetal blood into an Rh-negative mother tend to occur near the time of delivery. As a result, it is too late for the mother to become sensitized in time to transmit antibody to the infant before delivery. *(REF. 2 — p. 450)*

43. C. The long-acting sulfonamides interfere with the protein binding of bilirubin, which results in jaundice. *(REF. 2 — pp. 382, 443)*

44. C. Trisomy 18 is one of the more frequent chromosomal abnormalities associated with single umbilical artery. *(REF. 2 — p. 458)*

45. C. Facial erythema occurs and is frequently interpreted as a sign of good health and delays the seeking of medical attention. *(REF. 2 — p. 460)*

46. B. Withdrawal symptoms usually appear within 48 hours and are characterized by coarse tremors and hyperirritability. Other signs include tachypnea, diarrhea, vomiting, high-pitched cry and fever. Sneezing, yawning, nasal stuffiness and convulsions have been reported. *(REF. 2 — p. 463)*

47. D. Tetany is usually associated with transient hypoparathyroidism and not thyroid deficiency. *(REF. 2 — p. 464)*

48. E. Newborns with severe illnesses may develop hypoglycemia as a result of increased metabolic needs that are out of proportion to substrate stores and colonies provided. Hyperoxia by itself is not a stimulus for hypoglycemia. *(REF. 2 — pp. 466–467)*

49. A. Down's syndrome, meningomyelocele, and erythroblastosis fetalis can all be diagnosed by amniotic fluid analysis; however, achondroplasia cannot. *(REF. 1 — p. 125)*

50. B. Thalidomide and amphetamines have been shown conclusively to cause congenital malformations. Penicillin is not contraindicated during pregnancy. Insulin, when used appropriately, is not harmful to the fetus. *(REF. 2 — p. 381)*

51. E. If fetal tachycardia, flat baseline or late decelerations appear on the fetal monitor, then scalp capillary pH, $PaCO_2$, and base excess should be determined. Scalp pH should also be monitored in conditions such as preeclampsia that decrease placental transfer function. *(REF. 1 — p. 137)*

52. B. Duodenal and esophageal atresia are associated with polyhydramnios, whereas renal agenesis and pulmonary hypoplasia are associated with oligohydramnios. *(REF. 2 — p. 387)*

53. E. Pregnancies in which factors that increase the likelihood of abortion exist, fetal death, premature death, low birthweight, congenital malformations, mental retardation, or other handicapping conditions are termed high-risk pregnancies. *(REF. 2 — p. 387)*

54. C. The maternal urine estriol levels serve as a good index of placental function and are correlated with fetal size. They cannot be used to estimate gestational age or diagnose preeclampsia. *(REF. 1 — p. 131)*

55. B. Ultrasound can reliably determine crown rump length and biparietal diameter but is a poor predictor of fetal weight and cannot reliably determine the sex of the fetus. *(REF. 1 — p. 127)*

56. A. Intrauterine growth retardation is associated with maternal drug addiction, smoking, and malnutrition. Aspirin abuse is associated with neonatal platelet dysfunction but not growth retardation. *(REF. 1 — p. 173)*

57. D. Maternal anesthesia and analgesia can produce neurologically depressed infants and are not associated with neonatal jaundice or hyaline membrane disease. *(REF. 2 — pp. 380–382)*

58. B. Multiple births frequently produce infants with a difference in weight of 25% or greater. The mortality among multiple gestations is 7 times that of single births. Many twin births can occur vaginally without increased risk, but premature onset of labor is a frequent complication. *(REF. 1 — p. 170)*

II: Genetics

DIRECTIONS: Each of the questions or incomplete statements
below is followed by five suggested answers or completions. Select
the **one** that is **BEST** in each case.

59. In autosomal dominant inheritance the trait will be found in
    one parent and
    A. 25% of daughters and 75% of sons
    B. 25% of sons and 75% of daughters
  · C. 50% of daughters and 50% of sons
    D. only in daughters
    E. only in sons

60. Which of the following statements is NOT correct regarding
    X-linked inheritance?
  ⬂ A. Traits determined by genes carried on the X chromo-
       some may be either recessive or dominant in the female
    B. Traits determined by genes carried on the X chromo-
       some may be either recessive or dominant in the male
    C. A female may be heterozygous for an X-linked gene
    D. Recessive X-linked disorders are occasionally found in
       females who are homozygous for the disorder
    E. Males and females have X chromosomes

61. A human sperm contains
  ⬂ A. 23 pairs of chromosomes
    B. 46 chromosomes: 44 autosomes and two Y sex chromo-
       somes
    C. 46 chromosomes: 44 autosomes and X and Y chromo-
       somes
    D. 23 pairs of chromosomes and a Y sex chromosome
    E. 23 chromosomes: 22 autosomes and an X or a Y sex
       chromosome

20

62. The karyotype: 47, XX, + 21 represents a
    A. male with hermaphroditism
    ᵛ**B.** female with the Down's syndrome
    C. female with Klinefelter's syndrome
    D. female with mosaic for Turner's syndrome
    E. normal female

63. 46, XY, 18q⁻ describes a
    ᵛ**A.** male with deletion from the long arm of chromosome 18
    B. male with translocation from chromosome 18 to the Y
        chromosome
    C. male with Klinefelter's syndrome
    D. male with trisomy 18 syndrome
    E. normal male karyotype

64. Which of the following organs is probably the most sensitive
    to chromosomal imbalance?
    A. Brain
    B. Heart
    C. Kidney
    D. Eye
    E. Skeleton

65. It has been estimated that 5% to 10% of human conceptions
    have abnormal chromosomes. However, these defects are
    NOT detected in population surveys because
    A. clinical manifestations are not associated with abnormal
        chromosomes
    B. only trisomy states can be detected
    C. abnormal chromosomes do not produce a deficit unless
        they are translocated
    D. chromosome deficits cannot be detected until skeletal
        maturation is completed
    E. of none of the above

66. Turner's syndrome (45,X) is usually associated with all of the
    following EXCEPT
    ᵛ**A.** mental retardation
    B. short stature
    C. gonadal dysgenesis
    D. primary amenorrhea
    E. broad chest with widely spaced nipples

67. The characteristic karyotype in Klinefelter's syndrome is
    A. 46,XX, 46, XY
    ▸B. 47, XXY
    C. 48, XXX
    D. 46, Xi (Xg)
    E. 46, XY, 18g–

68. In a mating of two heterozygous persons for a recessive trait all of the following are correct EXCEPT
    A. 75% of the offspring appear phenotypically normal
    ‹B. 25% of the offspring are genotypically normal
    C. 50% of the children are heterozygous, like the parents
    D. the mother appears phenotypically abnormal
    E. the father appears phenotypically normal

69. If a person heterozygous for a recessive trait mates with a person heterozygous for the same recessive trait
    A. all of the children show the pathologic trait
    B. 75% of the offspring show the pathologic trait
    C. 50% of the offspring show the pathologic trait
    ˎ D. 25% of the offspring show the pathologic trait
    E. none of the offspring are affected

70. All of the following are inherited as dominant traits EXCEPT
    A. achondroplasia
    B. myotonia congenita
    C. tuberous sclerosis
    ▸D. cystic fibrosis
    E. osteogenesis imperfecta

71. The Barr body is
    A. an extra X chromosome in a male
    B. a projection of extra chromatin on an X chromosome
    C. a nonfunctional Y chromosome
    D. an extra Y chromosome
    ˎE. none of the above

72. All of the following statements regarding dermatoglyphic findings are correct EXCEPT
   A. in trisomy 21, excess ulnar loops are present and the radial loops are increased in fourth and fifth digits
   B. decreased arches on digits, usually less than three, multiple flexion crease on digits, and simian line are found in trisomy E (18) syndrome
   C. simian line, and arch fibular or arch fibular S pattern on hallucal area are found in trisomy D (13)
   D. increased whorls on fingers and an S hypothenar pattern are found in Turner's syndrome
   E. loops with low ridge counts on digits are characteristic of Klinefelter's syndrome

73. Trisomy 18 (Edwards' syndrome) is usually associated with all of the following EXCEPT
   A. mental retardation
   B. failure to thrive
   C. macrognathia
   D. low-set ears
   E. congenital heart disease

74. All of the following statements are correct concerning Down's syndrome EXCEPT
   A. prognosis for life is poor; most patients die by age 20 to 25 years
   B. males are generally sterile, females are fertile
   C. the average I.Q. is about 50; mental retardation is a prominent feature
   D. the children have a characteristic facies: flat nasal bridge, oblique palpebral fissure, flat occiput, and epicanthal folds
   E. trisomy 21 occurs in 95% of affected individuals

75. Which of the following illustrates the sex influence on autosomal inheritance?
   A. Pattern baldness
   B. Hemophilia
   C. Color blindness
   D. Xg blood group
   E. Glucose–6–phosphate dehydrogenase

76. All of the following are examples of human congenital defects due to the action of pleiotropic genes EXCEPT
    A. Down's syndrome with facial and cardiac anomalies
    B. Marfan's syndrome with anomalies of the eye, skeleton, and cardiovascular system
    C. osteogenesis imperfecta with blue sclera and otosclerosis
    D. acrocephalosyndactyly with abnormalities of skull and extremities
    E. mutation causing kidney agenesis and skeletal anomalies

77. Haploid gametes are derived from diploid cells of the gonad as a result of
    A. mitosis
    B. meiosis
    C. nondisjunction
    D. binary fission
    E. translocation

78. An XXXY male is studied cytogenetically. The anticipated number of Barr bodies is
    A. none
    B. one
    C. two
    D. three
    E. four

79. Skipping a generation is the rule in
    A. autosomal dominant inheritance
    B. autosomal recessive inheritance
    C. X-linked inheritance
    D. chromosomal defects (trisomy)
    E. none of the above

80. All of the following are inherited as dominant traits EXCEPT
    A. diabetes insipidus (ADH-deficient)
    B. ectodermal dysplasia (hydrotic)
    C. hemorrhagic telangiectasia
    D. Huntington's chorea
    E. Laurence-Moon-Biedl syndrome

81. If two persons who exhibit an abnormal recessive trait (bb)
    marry, the expected offspring are
    A. 75% normal, 25% abnormal
    B. 50% normal, 50% abnormal
    C. 25% abnormal, 75% normal
    D. 100% normal
    E. 100% abnormal

82. If a homozygous person with a pathologic trait mates with a
    normal person who is a heterozygous carrier of the same
    pathologic gene
    A. half of their children will appear normal, and half will ex-
       hibit the pathologic trait
    B. all of their children will be carriers of the pathologic trait,
       and none will look normal
    C. all of their children will exhibit the pathologic trait and
       appear abnormal
    D. one quarter will be abnormal carriers
    E. one quarter will be carriers and one quarter will be homo-
       zygous; half will be normal and will not carry the gene

83. All of the following are pathologic conditions inherited as
    autosomal recessives EXCEPT
    A. adrenogenital syndrome
    B. Morquio's disease
    C. Down's syndrome
    D. Niemann-Pick disease
    E. phenylketonuria

84. Which of the following is inherited as a sex-linked trait?
    A. Huntington's chorea
    B. Thalassemia minor
    C. Neurofibromatosis
    D. Myotonia congenita
    E. Progressive muscular dystrophy (Duchenne type)

85. Which of the following conditions is believed to depend on
    multiple genetic factors?
    A. Hartnup disease
    B. Morquio's disease
    C. Albinism
    D. Cleft lip and cleft palate
    E. Phenylketonuria

86. "Marker chromosomes" are
    A. associated with trisomy states
    B. representative of chromosomal deletions
    C. abnormally large chromosomes that cause lethal states
    D. pathologic states of the X chromosome observed in Turner's syndrome
    E. not pathognomonic of pathologic states

87. A human euploid cell can have the following chromosome number EXCEPT
    A. 46
    B. 69
    C. 92
    D. 108
    E. 138

88. 46 XY, 5p is the
    A. normal male karyotype
    B. male with the Down's syndrome
    C. cri-du-chat syndrome
    D. Turner's syndrome
    E. mosaic Klinefelter's syndrome

89. The incidence of Down's syndrome at maternal ages 45 years and older is approximately
    A. one in 2,000 births
    B. one in 1,000 births
    C. one in 600 births
    D. one in 250 births
    E. one in 50 births

90. Which of the following is NOT usually associated with trisomy 21?
    A. Hypertonia
    B. Brushfield spots
    C. Simian crease
    D. Congenital heart disease
    E. Flat nasal bridge

91. All of the following are usually associated with the cri-du-chat syndrome EXCEPT
    A. microcephaly
    B. round face
    C. mental retardation
    D. above average birthweight
    E. low-set malformed ears

92. Amniocentesis would probably NOT be recommended
    A. for routine determination of fetal sex
    B. when maternal age is over 40 years
    C. for known inherited translocation
    D. for prevention of X-linked recessive disorders
    E. because of a previous trisomic child

DIRECTIONS: Each set of lettered headings below is followed by a list of numbered words or phrases. For each numbered word or phrase select

    A if the item is associated with (A) *only*,
    B if the item is associated with (B) *only*,
    C if the item is associated with *both* (A) *and* (B),
    D if the item is associated with *neither* (A) *nor* (B).

    A. Cri-du-chat syndrome
    B. Down's syndrome
    C. Both
    D. Neither

93. Autosomal abnormality

94. Associated with an excess of chromosomal material

95. Can be caused by nondisjunction

96. Sex-linked abnormality

97. Caused by an abnormal chromosome number 5

Directions Summarized			
A	B	C	D
only	only	only	neither
A	B	A,B	A nor B

A. Turner's syndrome
B. Klinefelter's syndrome
C. Both
D. Neither

C 98. Associated with an abnormal number of X chromosomes

A 99. Sexual infantilism in adults

D 100. Seen in both sexes

D 101. Severe mental retardation is characteristic

D 102. Can be diagnosed without a karyotype

A. Hemophilia A
B. Sickle cell anemia
C. Both
D. Neither

D 103. Inherited as an autosomal disorder

D 104. All sons of the affected male will also be affected

A 105. If one parent is affected then the chance for having an affected child is 50%

A 106. All daughters of an affected father will be carriers

A 107. Expression of the disease can skip generations in a family

A. Trisomy 18
B. Trisomy 13
C. Both
D. Neither

C 108. Associated with severe developmental delay

109. More common in live-born infants than trisomy 21

110. Survival is common to third decade of life

111. May have cleft lip

112. Abnormalities of the hands commonly found

II: Genetics
Answers and Comments

59. C. Autosomal dominant inheritance indicates that the trait is not sex-linked. In a mating in which a parent passes either a normal or a mutant gene to the offspring and the corresponding genes derived from the other parent are normal, 50% of the children will be normal and 50% (male or female) will exhibit the trait: *(REF. 1 — p. 271)*

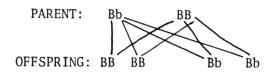

60. B. In the male, who has only *one* X chromosome, a trait will always be expressed. Whereas a female can be heterozygous or homozygous for an X-linked gene the male can only be homozygous. An X-linked recessive gene in a female is always clinically manifested in the male. *(REF. 1 — p. 273)*

61. E. The germ cells, in this case the sperm, have 23 chromosomes, i.e., one member of each pair. This is the haploid number of chromosomes: 22 autosomes and one sex chromosome (either X or Y). *(REF. 1 — p. 279)*

62. B. The karyotype cited indicates an extra chromosome (number 21) in a female (XX) with Down's syndrome (trisomy 21). *(REF. 1 — p. 280)*

63. A. 46 designates the normal number of chromosomes and XY indicates a male. The designation 18q⁻ pertains to the deletion from the long arm of chromosome 18. *(REF. 1 — p. 281)*

64. A. The brain and the sex organs are probably the most sensitive to disruptions in chromosome balance. Mental retardation is a common sequela of chromosomal abnormality. *(REF. 1 — p. 285)*

65. E. The reason we do not see the expected 5% to 10% of an involved population with these defects is that approximately 95% are spontaneously aborted. *(REF. 1 — p. 285)*

66. A. Mental retardation is *not* a characteristic feature of Turner's syndrome (unlike the other syndromes associated with abnormalities of chromosome number). Mental retardation appears in less than 10% of patients with Turner's syndrome. Academic underachievement may be associated with the visual motor perceptual problems found in patients with Turner's syndrome. *(REF. 1 — p. 286)*

67. B. The characteristic karyotype is 47, XXY, which indicates an extra chromosome, X, in the genetic makeup. Variants have been described: 48, XXXY, and 49, XXXXY. *(REF. 1 — p. 286)*

68. D. All statements are correct except D.

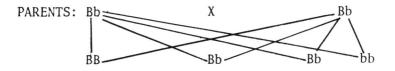

75%: **BB, Bb, Bb** = phenotypically normal
25%: **BB** = genotypically normal
50%: **Bb, Bb** = heterozygous like the parents

Both the mother and father are carriers of the recessive gene but appear phenotypically normal. *(REF. 2 — p. 340)*

69. D. 25% of the offspring are affected, i.e., each child has one chance in four of being homozygous and having the pathologic trait. *(REF. 2 — p. 340)*

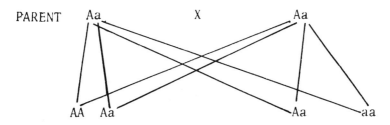

70. D. All of the pathologic conditions listed are inherited as autosomal dominant traits, except for cystic fibrosis. Cystic fibrosis is inherited as an autosomal recessive trait. *(REF. 2 — p. 339)*

71. E. The Barr body is the sex-chromatin body characteristic of female somatic nuclei. In the normal female, one X chromosome replicates its DNA during mitosis later than the other chromosomes and remains inactive in the interphase cell. *(REF. 2 — pp. 340–341)*

72. B. The findings associated with trisomy E or trisomy 18 syndrome include excess arches on digits (more than six), simian line, and single flexion crease on digits. *(REF. 1 — p. 292)*

73. C. Micrognathia is associated with trisomy 18 syndrome. The micrognathia has been termed "fish mouth" by some investigators. *(REF. 1 — p. 288)*

74. A. All of the statements are true, except for the comment regarding prognosis for life. Prognosis is fairly good for a life expectancy of 30 to 50 years. Major factors to be considered are the complications of leukemia and congenital heart disease. The patients are also more susceptible to infection. However, modern therapy has improved the life expectancy. *(REF. 1 — pp. 287–288)*

75. A. Pattern baldness is determined by an autosomal gene. However, it acts as a dominant trait in men and as a recessive trait in women. *(REF. 1 — p. 273)*

76. A. The anomalies associated with Down's syndrome are *not* the result of a pleiotropic effect of a gene mutation but rather of a chromosomal abnormality (trisomy 21). *(REF. 1 — p. 277)*

77. B. Meiosis, or reduction division, is a process during which the homologous chromosomes pair up and then divide. As a result of the separation, one member of the pair goes to one daughter cell and the other to the opposite daughter cell. If the diploid number of chromosomes were 46, the haploid cell would contain 23 chromosomes. *(REF. 3 — p. 289)*

78. C. The Barr body is a sex-chromatin body observed in the interphase nucleus. It represents an X chromosome replicating DNA late in mitosis. It remains as discrete, condensed, physiologically inactive chromatin mass. The number of Barr bodies is one less than the number of X chromosomes in the diploid complement. In the case of XXXY there would be two Barr bodies. *(REF. 2 — p. 365)*

79. E. Skipping a generation is not a fixed rule. It may occur as a result of reduced gene expressivity, causing less apparent clinical manifestations. Skipping a generation may also be seen as a result of reduced penetrance in which there is no expression of the abnormal gene. *(REF. 2 — pp. 338, 340, 341)*

80. E. The only disorder on this list that is *not* inherited as a dominant trait is Laurence-Moon-Biedl syndrome. This disorder is inherited as an autosomal recessive trait. *(REF. 2 — p. 339)*

81. E. It is readily apparent that all of the offspring will be abnormal. *(REF. 2 — p. 340)*

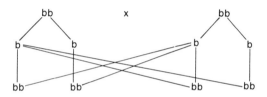

82. A. Half of the children will be normal in appearance and half will exhibit the pathologic trait. The schema below indicates the inheritance pattern. *(REF. 2 — p. 340)*

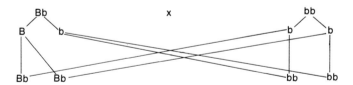

83. C. All of the conditions cited are inherited as autosomal recessive traits except Down's syndrome. This represents a chromosomal abnormality, trisomy 21 or a 21 translocation. *(REF. 2 — p. 339)*

84. E. All of the conditions cited are inherited as autosomal dominant traits except progressive muscular dystrophy (Duchenne type), which is a sex-linked trait. *(REF. 2 — p. 339)*

85. D. All of the disorders listed, except cleft lip and cleft palate, are manifestations of single-gene autosomal recessive inheritance.

Cleft lip and cleft palate do not conform to the established patterns of Mendelian inheritance. They may represent the effect of several involved genes. *(REF. 2 — pp. 339, 342)*

86. E. "Marker chromosomes" are normal morphologic variants found in normal karyotypes, e.g., elongation of the centromere region of chromosome numbers 1, 9, and 16. They do not represent pathologic states. *(REF. 2 — pp. 345, 346)*

87. D. All of the chromosome complements are correct. A euploid cell is an exact multiple of the haploid number. In humans the haploid number is 23, therefore 46, 69, and 92 are all euploid cells. The diploid number is 46, and 69, 92, and 138 are polyploid cells. *(REF. 2 — p. 347)*

88. C. The karyotype cited indicates a male with the normal number of chromosomes (46) but with a deletion of the short arm of chromosome 5. This represents cat-cry (cri-du-chat) syndrome. *(REF. 2 — p. 349)*

89. E. The incidence in the general population of Down's syndrome (trisomy 21 syndrome) is one in 600 to 700 births. The incidence increases with advancing maternal age. In mothers over 45 years, the incidence rises to one in 50 births. The reason for the correlation between late maternal age and nondisjunction is still unknown. *(REF. 2 — pp. 352–353)*

90. A. Hypotonia is usually associated with trisomy 21, Down's syndrome. Hypertonia is more characteristic of the trisomy 18 syndrome. *(REF. 2 — p. 355)*

91. D. Cri-du-chat syndrome is associated with low birthweight, which is characteristic of most deletion syndromes. All of the other characteristics cited are observed with cat-cry syndrome. *(REF. 2 — p. 358)*

92. A. Although the risk associated with amniocentesis is small, it is not recommended for routine fetal sex determination. Priority is given to more significant areas of concern involving genetic and chromosomal faults. *(REF. 2 — p. 369)*

93. C. Both Down's syndrome and cri-du-chat syndrome are
94. B. autosomal abnormalities. Down's has an excess of genetic

95. A. material while cri-du-chat has a deletion of the short arm
96. D. of chromosome 5. Neither syndrome is sex-linked. *(REF.*
97. A. *2 — p. 347)*

98. C. Turner's and Klinefelter's syndromes are disorders caused
99. A. by the presence of an abnormal number of X chromo-
100. D. somes (Turner's too few, Klinefelter's too many). Turner's
101. D. patients have the female phenotype and are sexually in-
102. D. fantile adults, while those with Klinefelter's are males who
develop secondary sex characteristics. Although buccal
smears can suggest the diagnosis, a karyotype is mandatory. Severe
mental retardation is not seen in either condition *(REF. 1 — p. 286)*

103. B. Sickle cell anemia and hemophilia A are recessive dis-
104. D. eases, the expression of which can skip generations. The
105. A. daughters of a father with the sex-linked recessive dis-
106. A. order will all be carriers, and one half of his children
107. C. (males) will have the disease. Sickle cell anemia is an autosomal disorder, and the sex of offspring does not affect
inheritance. *(REF. 1 — p. 293)*

108. C. Trisomy 13 and 18 are two very similar autosomal abnor-
109. D. malities. Both are associated with developmental delay,
110. D. cleft lip, anomalies of the hands, and death in early in-
111. C. fancy. Neither is more common than Down's syndrome.
112. C. *(REF. 1 — p. 289)*

III: Developmental and Behavioral Pediatrics

DIRECTIONS: Each of the questions or incomplete statements below is followed by five suggested answers or completions. Select the **one** that is **BEST** in each case.

113. Which of the following developmental landmarks is usually NOT observed when examining a four-month-old?
    A. Infant laughs
    B. Responsive smiles
    C. Eyes follow object for 180°
    D. Transferral of block from one hand to another
    E. Holds head erect when held in a sitting position

114. You are called to see the mother of a two-day-old newborn. She is extremely anxious because she has discovered a darkly pigmented area over the baby's sacrum and buttocks. The most likely diagnosis is
    A. malignant melanoma
    B. erythema toxicum
    C. mongolian spot
    D. port-wine stain
    E. meningomyelocele

115. The mother of a two-month-old baby is very much concerned because her baby sleeps too much. The history indicates that the infant is not sleeping excessively. The norm for a two-month-old is about
    A. ten to 12 hours/day
    B. 12 to 14 hours/day
    C. 14 to 15 hours/day
    D. 15 to 18 hours/day
    E. more than 20 hours/day

116. All of the following are characteristic of colic EXCEPT
    A. crying is the cardinal manifestation
    B. legs are held as if the infant is experiencing pain
    C. eructation and flatus are common
    D. etiology is unknown
    E. usually starts at age four months and lasts two to three months

117. A three-year-old child is usually NOT able to
    A. climb stairs with alternating feet
    B. draw a person with five parts
    C. know his/her sex
    D. give his/her full name
    E. copy a circle

118. The Denver Developmental Screening Test (DDST) is valuable in assessing all of the following EXCEPT
    A. gross motor development
    B. fine motor development
    C. reading
    D. language
    E. social development

119. A four-year-old child refuses to eat (anorexia). Careful examination indicates this is a behavior problem. Treatment includes all of the following EXCEPT
    A. do not offer food between meal times
    B. place food before child without fanfare; he can eat or not eat without comment
    C. discontinue bribing or other tricks to encourage eating
    D. attempt a trial of a mild appetite stimulant
    E. do not overexaggerate the situation; counsel the anxious parents

120. All of the following are characteristic of psychogenic vomiting EXCEPT
    A. it is usually not seen until after six years of age
    B. it is not associated with food hypersensitivity
    C. in school age child it may be associated with school phobia
    D. it can be confused with vomiting due to expanding intracranial lesions
    E. it may require psychotherapy

121. A seven-year-old boy was bowel and bladder trained at four years of age. At age six enuresis occurred, which coincided with the birth of a sibling. The bed-wetting could be caused by all of the following EXCEPT
    A. diabetes mellitus
    B. cystitis
    C. birth of the sibling
    D. too liberal a TV-viewing schedule
    E. organic problems

122. A two-year-child exhibits restlessness and disturbed sleep. Physical examination reveals no abnormalities. Crying persists until a parent turns on the room light and plays with the child. The best therapy is
    A. to allow the child to come to his parents' bed
    B. to continue playing with the child until he is very sleepy
    C. to spank child and allow him to cry
    D. to feed the child warm milk and cookies
    E. to initiate a sound behavior modification program

123. Imipramine is effective in enuresis because it
    A. relaxes the bladder
    B. tenses the urethral sphincter
    C. causes renal slowdown
    D. depresses the hypothalamus
    E. influences the physiology of sleep

124. Head-banging
    A. usually occurs in children three to five years of age
    B. usually occurs in midafternoon
    C. is always associated with mental retardation
    D. is best treated with diazepam
    E. usually requires no major therapeutic intervention

125. Finger-sucking in a three-year-old is best treated by
    A. binding the hand in a mitten
    B. applying a pepper solution to the fingers
    C. restraining hand behind the back
    D. spanking when observed finger-sucking
    E. a conservative approach with reduction of parental anxieties

126. Mutism in a three-year-old is most likely caused by
   A. congenital or early acquired deafness
   B. mental retardation
   C. hysteria
   D. negativism
   E. severe chorea

127. Truancy differs from school phobia in that the truant
   A. is usually hyperkinetic and has a short attention span
   B. is almost always a male juvenile delinquent
   C. absents himself from school and home
   D. fears examinations and report cards
   E. usually has a history of autistic behaviors

128. The average vocabulary of a two-year-old American, of middle-class background, is approximately
   A. 75 words
   B. 125 words
   C. 175 words
   D. 200 words
   E. more than 200 words

129. Which of the following is probably of LEAST importance in regulating the behavior of a six-week-old baby?
   A. Tactile stimulation
   B. Kinesthetic impulses
   C. Thermal changes
   D. Visual impulses
   E. Olfactory sensation

130. The most common cause of short stature associated with delayed sexual development is a result of
   A. primordial dwarfism
   B. maternal deprivation and child abuse
   C. hypothyroidism
   D. deletion of the short arm of chromosome number 3
   E. constitutional delayed growth

131. Hypoxia affects growth in a manner similar to
    A. caloric deprivation
    B. dwarfism
    C. constitutional delayed growth
    D. maternal deprivation
    E. allergy

132. The most universal cause of growth retardation is
    A. hypoxia secondary to congenital heart disease
    B. malnutrition
    C. repeated respiratory infections
    D. maternal deprivation
    E. chromosomal abnormalities

133. During the process of normal adolescent growth and development, male gynecomastia is associated with all of the following EXCEPT
    A. it occurs at midpuberty in about 50% of boys
    B. it is usually a transient phenomenon
    C. it usually resolves spontaneously within 18 months
    D. it is usually treated effectively with corticosteroids
    E. it may be of significant psychologic concern

134. The first sign of puberty in a normal male is usually the
    A. increase in size of the testes
    B. appearance of facial hair
    C. appearance of axillary hair
    D. appearance of pubic hair
    E. appearance of body hair

135. In the United States, the average age of menarche is approximately
    A. nine to ten years
    B. ten and one half to 11 1/2 years
    C. 12 1/2 to 13 years
    D. 14 to 15 years
    E. 15 to 17 1/2 years

136. Radiographic examination to determine skeletal maturity is best evaluated by x-rays of the
   A. elbow joint
   B. wrist
   C. ankle
   D. knee joint
   E. hip

137. You are asked to evaluate the developmental status of a one-year-old child. The child cannot sit without support. He can grasp with one hand. He can say "baba" and "dada"; he responds to "no". However, he cannot understand the names of objects and does not show interest in pictures. The child does not creep, cannot stand holding on, and cannot use finger-thumb apposition to pick up small objects. He can transfer objects from hand to hand. These observations suggest the child is
   A. mentally retarded, profound level
   B. mentally retarded, severe-moderate level
   C. functioning at a six- to eight-month level
   D. functioning at an 11-month level
   E. functioning at age level

138. A seven-year-old child has had no problems until he begins school and has to repeat the first grade. No diagnostic evaluation has been performed. The diagnosis may be any of the following EXCEPT
   A. mild mental retardation
   B. unrecognized seizure state
   C. progressive degenerative neurologic disease
   D. problem is of no concern; the child is "a late bloomer"
   E. previously undetected organic handicap such as a hearing loss

139. Which of the following is pathognomonic of attentional deficit disorder?
   A. Soft neurologic signs
   B. Characteristic EEG changes
   C. Psychologic evaluation
   D. Type of specific learning disabilities
   E. None of the above

140. Mild mental retardation is suggested by an I.Q. between
   A. 80 and 90
   B. 20 and 40
   C. 50 and 70
   D. 40 and 50
   E. below 30

141. A four-year-old is suspected of being mentally retarded. Which of the following would be useful in determining the child's I.Q.?
   A. Boehm Test of Basic Concepts
   B. Denver Developmental Screening Test
   C. Meeting Street School Screening Test
   D. Gesell Developmental Scales
   E. None of the above

142. Which of the following comments does NOT apply to the Stanford-Binet Intelligence Scale?
   A. Can be used from age two years to adult
   B. Yields a mental age and intelligence quotient
   C. Can correlate with school achievement
   D. Some elements of cultural bias
   E. An exam heavily weighted with visual items

143. Which of the following controversial programs, claiming to assist learning in handicapped children, is based on a theory suggesting that phylogeny recapitulates ontogeny and that skills must be learned in a sequence that is logical in order to promote adequate functioning?
   A. Ayres' sensory integrative approach
   B. Frostig program of visual perception
   C. Doman-Delacato neurologic organization
   D. Optometric exercising
   E. Food additive diet

144. Which of the following examinations has a high predictive value in identifying a preschooler with specific learning disabilities?
   A. Denver Developmental Screening Test
   B. Thematic Apperception Test
   C. Peabody Picture Vocabulary Test
   D. Stanford-Binet Intelligence Scales
   E. None of the examinations cited are of high predictive value

145. Concerning adoption
    A. statistics reveal that most adopted children and their families do *not* adjust well
    B. private adoptions are preferred over agency adoptions
    C. the best age for adoption is eight months of age
    D. adopted children should be told of the adoption at about three years of age
    E. adopted children should *not* be told of the adoption

146. The peak incidence of temper tantrums in children is
    A. before one year of age
    B. around two and one half years of age
    C. about age four years
    D. between six and eight years of age
    E. over ten years of age

147. A two and a half-year-old child is enrolled in a day-care center. Which of the following psychological adjustments is anticipated?
    A. The child will exhibit separation anxieties, fears, and apprehensions that will cause hyperkinesis
    B. The child will regress in areas of speech and language
    C. The long-range effect will be maternal rejection by the child
    D. The child-mother relationship suffers, and both will have a tense relationship with "nervous" habits
    E. None of the above are documented statements

148. All of the following are characteristic of pica EXCEPT
    A. it occurs most often during the first three years of life
    B. it has been observed commonly in mentally retarded children
    C. it may be associated with neurotic children
    D. it may represent a mineral or vitamin deficiency
    E. therapy requires the use of repeated forced emesis following discovery of ingestion of any item as a behavior modification approach

149. Breath-holding is characterized by all of the following EX-CEPT
   A. it may be similar to a temper tantrum
   B. it may be seen in young infants when startled
   C. in severe cases there may be a momentary loss of consciousness
   D. symptoms may result from hypoxia
   E. at the height of attack, the child should be disciplined

150. Anorexia nervosa
   A. is more common in preadolescent boys
   B. is characterized by reigning starvation without weight loss
   C. is associated with low standards, loose superegos, and apathetic personalities
   D. is most frequently observed in low economic groups
   E. requires psychotherapy

151. Autism (as originally described by Kanner) is characterized by all of the following EXCEPT
   A. loss of contact with people
   B. obsession for sameness
   C. strong (affectionate) relationship to inanimate objects
   D. good response to methylphenidate
   E. there is no readily available drug therapy

152. Children with learning disorders should receive a therapeutic trial of
   A. dextroamphetamine
   B. methylphenidate
   C. pemoline
   D. diphenhydramine
   E. medications are *not* indicated

III: Developmental and Behavioral Pediatrics Answers and Comments

113. D. A four-month-old is capable of all of the milestones cited except for transfer of objects from one hand to another. This skill is probably not developed until the child is approximately eight to nine months of age. *(REF. 1 — p. 24)*

114. C. The description most closely resembles that of a mongolian spot. The mother should be reassured that this is a benign condition. The spot usually fades and disappears during the first year of life. *(REF. 1 — p. 28)*

115. D. During the first three months of life an infant averages 15 to 18 hours of sleep daily; the range is 13 to 20 hours. The periods of sleep vary from two to four hours. The total sleep time is variable. *(REF. 1 — p. 29)*

116. E. Colic tends to appear during the first few months of infancy and rarely lasts past four months of life. The crying is often intense and inconsolable. Family support is essential, since colic can cause stress. *(REF. 1 — p. 30)*

117. B. A three-year-old is capable of performing all of the tasks except drawing a person with five parts. At age three years the drawing would probably be a circle, with little resemblance to a human face. At age four to five years the drawing probably would contain four or five recognizable parts; at age five to six years about eight recognizable parts or details. *(REF. 1 — p. 35)*

118. C. The DDST is a good screening inventory of development from birth through age six years. It does not assess reading skills. *(REF. 1 — p. 69)*

119. D. Refusal of food is one of the most common behavior problems in children between two and five years of age. Treatment as suggested is a valuable part of a counseling program with parents avoiding medicines and food supplements. Early counseling is a helpful preventative measure. *(REF. 1 — p. 79)*

120. A. Psychogenic vomiting can occur at any age. It may be a symptom of emotional maladjustment or a serious neurotic disorder. *(REF. 1 — p. 79)*

121. D. All of the etiologies listed are possible causes of secondary enuresis except the TV habits. Although the birth of the sibling appears to be an obvious cause, organic etiologies must be ruled out. *(REF. 1 — p. 80)*

122. E. None of the first four therapies listed are psychologically sound. Providing the child with company will *not* break the habit. An investigation is in order, followed by parent counseling and behavior modification. *(REF. 1 — p. 81)*

123. E. Imipramine probably exerts its effect on nocturnal enuresis by increasing lighter non-rapid eye movement sleep and decreasing rapid eye movement, or dream sleep. *(REF. 1 — p. 81)*

124. E. Head-banging occurs in perfectly normal children. It is seen usually between six and 12 months of age, occurs usually at bedtime, and, for the most part, runs a benign course and stops without therapy. *(REF. 1 — p. 82)*

125. E. The child should be kept busy with other things, and the parent should be reassured. When associated with general immaturity in an older child, careful study is indicated. *(REF. 1 — p. 83)*

126. A. Mutism is usually related to deafness. The other causes listed are possible but are not as common as deafness. Deafness must always be considered in any form of language disorder. *(REF. 1 — p. 84)*

127. C. The child with school phobia refuses to go to school and elects to stay at home. The truant may go off to school, cuts class, and does *not* return home. Truancy is most frequent in adolescents, whereas school phobia occurs early in a child's school career. Truancy may reflect poor academic adjustment, improper class placement, or poor self-concept. *(REF. 1 — p. 87)*

128. E. The average American, middle-class child at age two years usually has a vocabulary of at least 300 words. At this age words are combined to make meaningful sentences. *(REF. 1 — p. 257)*

129. D. In a six-week-old baby, vision is probably the least important regulator of behavior. Vision does not become important until binocular fixation has been stabilized; this probably occurs during the fourth month of life. *(REF. 1 — p. 254)*

130. E. The most common cause of short stature and delayed sexual development is constitutional delayed growth. *(REF. 1 — p. 249)*

131. A. Hypoxia has an effect similar to caloric deprivation, and is characterized by failure to multiply muscle cells or by poor protein synthesis. *(REF. 1 — p. 648)*

132. B. Malnutrition is the most universal cause of growth retardation. Depending on the type of malnutrition, growth can be retarded either by diminished cell size or as a result of decreased cell multiplication. *(REF. 1 — p. 248)*

133. D. All of the other statements regarding male gynecomastia in adolescence are correct. The gynecomastia is usually of great concern to the male adolescent and counseling is necessary to stress the transient nature of this phenomenon. Steroids are not recommended for this condition. *(REF. 1 — p. 241)*

134. A. The appearance of pubic hair growth usually follows the increase in size of the testes, which coincides with the onset of the adolescent growth (height) spurt. Facial, body, and axillary hair usually appear approximately two years after the growth of pubic hair. *(REF. 1 — p. 241)*

135. C. In the U.S., the age of onset of menarche has been decreasing by approximately four months per decade since 1840. Menarche commences approximately at ages 12 ½ to 13 years of age. *(REF. 1 — p. 240)*

136. B. The hand and the wrist are the preferred sites for several reasons: 1) convenience, 2) variety and number of developing bones present, and 3) the information documented about this area. *(REF. 1 — p. 240)*

137. C. The milestones that this child has achieved correspond to those of a child six to eight months of age. At one year, he should be able to stand holding on, walk with support, say two to three words with meaning, and understand names of objects. The label, mental retardation, cannot be applied until more data are available; for example, can the child see and hear? Although delays in multiple areas suggest mental retardation, the child requires more extensive diagnostic evaluation. In essence, a level of functional ability is designated but more data is required before classification is attempted. *(REF. 1 — p. 1734)*

138. D. The child may have any one of the disorders listed; conditions that need not have obvious manifestations during the preschool period. To the list could be added, attentional deficit disorder, specific learning disabilities (perceptual problems) or previously undetected vision and hearing loss. The diagnosis of "late bloomer," or maturational lag *without* investigation of other possibilities is not recommended. *(REF. 1 — p. 1736)*

139. E. There are no pathognomonic signs of attentional deficit disorder. The diagnosis is based on cumulative data from history and physical and psychologic evaluation. The disorder may be suggested by the complex of symptoms: hyperactivity, short attention span, impulsivity, distractibility, and school failure despite average intelligence. *(REF. 1 — pp. 1764-1765)*

140. C. Mild mental retardation (I.Q. 50 to 70 as per the American Association of Mental Deficiency) indicates that the individual is educable, probably to a third to fifth grade level. Individuals so affected have some degree of independence in daily living. *(REF. 1 — p. 1767)*

141. E. None of the screening tests listed are of value in I.Q. determinations. They are *all* screening tests and should not be used to assess an intelligence quotient. Probably the best test to use for a 4-year-old would be the Stanford Binet Intelligence Scale or the Wechsler Pre-School and Primary Scale of Infant Intelligence. *(REF. 1 — pp. 1786-1787)*

142. E. By about age six this examination is verbally oriented and it may penalize the child with learning problems. The examination is not grouped into verbal and performance subtests. *(REF. 1 — p. 1787)*

143. C. The Doman-Delacato theory suggests that when a dysfunction is apparent, the therapy program requires relearning at an earlier stage. The program requires motor-patterning procedures, and it is controversial and has not been recognized by several official medical groups. *(REF. 1 — p. 1799)*

144. E. At the present time there is no single examination, or test battery, that has good predictive value for detecting the preschooler who will have difficulty in school. General intelligence can be assessed, but identification of specific learning disabilities cannot. Perceptual norms for preschoolers have not been well defined. *(REF. 1 — p. 1791)*

145. D. All of the other statements are incorrect. The adopted child should be told of the adoption when he has developed verbal skills and comprehension, usually between ages three and four years. The child will probably require multiple repetitions and explanations of the adoption, in particular settings and circumstances. The explanations should not be difficult to comprehend or too ritualized a procedure. *(REF. 2 — p. 76)*

146. B. Temper tantrums are not uncommon and reach their peak incidence at about age two and a half years. Often they serve the child as an attention-seeking mechanism. In modifying this behavior, attempts are made to indicate that the temper tantrum is a useless behavior that does not gather rewards. *(REF. 2 — p. 71)*

147. E. There have been no documented evidences to suggest the development of pathologic states when a young child attends a day-care program of good quality. Depending on the circumstances, the utilization of a day-care program may have numerous beneficial ramifications for child and parent. The key is the regulation of good, qualified, and well-staffed day-care programs. *(REF. 2 — p. 73)*

148. E. The behavior modification for pica is *not* this forceful and negative an approach. Therapy is directed toward providing the child with adequate measures for satisfying the oral stage of development, e.g., sucking, biting, chewing, etc. *(REF. 2 — p. 89)*

149. E. The child cannot be disciplined during the attack because he has a temporary loss of objectivity. Punishment is usually not effective in handling breath-holding. The child requires understanding, reassurance, and kindness. Finding methods of prevention is the challenge. *(REF. 2 — p. 98)*

150. E. Anorexia nervosa is more commonly observed in adolescent girls who have strict superegos and high standards and achievement levels for themselves. The condition may be precipitated by mild criticisms or challenges. The intense starvation causes severe weight loss. Psychotherapy is indicated. *(REF. 2 — pp. 88-89)*

151. D. Autism is often manifested by regression, rocking motions, and mutism; intelligence appears to be intact. The differential diagnosis includes mental retardation, agnosia, aphasia, deafness, and neurologic degeneration. Methylphenidate has not been recommended in the therapy of autism. *(REF. 2 — pp. 112-113)*

152. E. At best, medication is an adjunct in treating children with learning disabilities. The program usually requires educational planning, counseling, and special education resources. Medicines do *not* cause learning. *(REF. 2 — p. 151)*

IV: Accidents, Poisonings, and Environmental Hazards

DIRECTIONS: Each of the questions or incomplete statements below is followed by five suggested answers or completions. Select the one that is BEST in each case.

153. Which of the following statements regarding childhood accidents is FALSE?
    A. The majority of injuries in children of all age groups are sustained in the home
    B. From birth to 14 years of age, motor vehicle accidents rank first among fatal accidents
    C. Among children one through four years, deaths are primarily caused by fire, burns, and explosions
    D. Accidents occur more frequently among boys than girls
    E. Some children are accident-prone, and accidents cannot be prevented in this group

154. Concerning the incidence, epidemiology, and etiology of drowning in children, all of the following are true EXCEPT
    A. boys are more prone to such accidents than girls
    B. death is caused by asphyxia with fluid aspiration
    C. CNS damage may become irreversible within three to seven minutes after the beginning of immersion and within less than one minute after cardiocirculatory arrest
    D. consciousness and absence of apnea are synonymous with recovery
    E. presence of breathing movements and coughing when child is removed from the water suggests that hypoxic damage and aspiration are probably slight

155. The most common cause of burns in children is related to
   A. low-voltage household electrical current
   B. flammable clothing
   C. scalding by spilling or immersion
   D. chemically strong acids
   E. contact with high-voltage wires

156. Which of the following statements is true of a second-degree leg burn sustained by a five-year-old child?
   A. The use of hexachlorophene as a cleansing agent is contraindicated
   B. routinely, the burned area is covered with a topical antibiotic
   C. the child should be given hyperimmune human antitetanus serum
   D. Routine administration of an oral broad-spectrum antibiotic is recommended
   E. Immediate hospitalization is required

157. Approximately 44% of all poisonings in children are a result of
   A. the ingestion of drugs intended for internal medication
   B. the ingestion of household chemicals
   C. the ingestion of berries and leaves of poisonous plants
   D. the eating of poisonous and contaminated foods
   E. the inhalation of toxic solvents

158. A child with gastroenteritis, stupor, convulsions, and circulatory collapse was reported to have ingested "something from a plant." The most suspicious plant would be
   A. seeds of larkspur
   B. flowers of oleander
   C. seeds of jimsonweed
   D. castor beans and seeds
   E. leaves of azalea

159. Gastric lavage is contraindicated after ingestion of
   A. aspirin
   B. corrosive alkali
   C. diazepam
   D. castor beans
   E. vitamins

160. A four-year-old has confirmed salicylate toxicity. The first sign is usually
    A. petechiae and gingival bleeding
    B. diplopia and peripheral blindness
    C. hyperventilation
    D. diarrhea and vomiting
    E. convulsions

161. A two-year-old child has ingested toxic amounts of iron (as an oral hematinic). The first sign to be noted within the first hour is
    A. vomiting and bloody diarrhea
    B. tremors, convulsions, and coma
    C. hyperventilation
    D. petechiae and bleeding from the gums
    E. hallucinations

162. The toxicity of petroleum distillates is related to
    A. aspiration of hydrocarbon into the respiratory tract
    B. gastric ulceration and hemorrhage
    C. CNS depression, convulsions, and coma
    D. renal parenchyma destruction and renal failure
    E. hemolysis of red blood cells and hemoglobinuria

163. An 18-year-old has been mainlining heroin (intravenous administration). All of the following are expected EXCEPT
    A. relative oliguria
    B. increase in body temperature
    C. euphoria and pain relief
    D. miosis
    E. minimal effects on cardiovascular system

164. An adolescent presents to an emergency room in coma, with constricted pupils, respiratory depression, cyanosis, and rales. The most likely diagnosis is
    A. bilateral bronchopneumonia
    B. acute heroin toxicity
    C. acute amphetamine toxicity
    D. an LSD trip
    E. too much whiskey

165. The most commonly abused pharmacological agent(s) is/are
    A. marijuana and barbiturates
    B. LSD
    C. cocaine
    D. heroin
    E. alcohol

166. In which of the following age groups is the incidence of drowning highest?
    A. 10-19 years
    B. 3-5 years
    C. 5-7 years
    D. 7-10 years
    E. 1-3 years

167. In approximately what percentage of drowning victims is aspiration NOT a cause of death?
    A. 50%
    B. 10%
    C. 75%
    D. 2%
    E. 0.5%

168. In the U.S., how many deaths are annually attributed to drowning?
    A. 5,000 to 6,000
    B. 200 to 400
    C. 6,000 to 10,000
    D. 1,000 to 2,000
    E. 25,000 to 30,000

169. All of the following are characteristic of food poisoning by *Clostridium botulinum* EXCEPT
    A. occurrence of central nervous system symptoms within two to four hours
    B. diagnosis may be confirmed by serologic demonstration of toxin in blood
    C. specific antitoxin is available
    D. death may occur in one to eight days
    E. triad of absence of pupillary reflex, dry, rough tongue surface, and respiratory paralysis is characteristic

170. Causative exotoxins have been demonstrated for
    A. *Staphylococcus aureus*
    B. *Streptococcus faecalis*
    C. *Escherichia coli*
    D. *Pseudomonas enteritis*
    E. all forms of viral gastroenteritis

171. In the U.S., the relative rank of accidents and poisonings as a cause of death in the pediatric age group is
    A. first
    B. second
    C. fourth
    D. sixth
    E. seventh

172. Which one of the following is the most frequent cause of poisoning in children less than five years of age?
    A. Insecticides
    B. Floor polish
    C. Tranquilizers
    D. Aspirin
    E. Turpentine

173. Some poisons have characteristic actions; for example, dilated pupils may be caused by all of the following EXCEPT
    A. atropine
    B. ephedrine
    C. muscarine
    D. nicotine (late)
    E. cocaine

174. Methemoglobinemia can be caused by all of the following EXCEPT
    A. nitrites
    B. aniline derivatives
    C. acetanilid
    D. phenazopyridine HCl
    E. chloral hydrate

175. An accidental poisoning of a three-year-old child has occurred 20 minutes before he is seen in an emergency room.
The suspected poison is strychnine. What course of action
should be taken?
    A. Gastric lavage with 200 ml of 1:5,000 potassium
    permanganate
    B. Gastric lavage with 150 ml of saline
    C. Gastric lavage with 200 ml of weak salt and sodium
    bicarbonate
    D. Gastric lavage with 250 ml of distilled water
    E. Gastric lavage may not be indicated

176. A two-year-old child has ingested 30 ml of methyl alcohol.
All of the following are correct EXCEPT
    A. toxic and degenerative changes occur in the liver, kid-
    ney, brain, and heart
    B. formic acid or formaldehyde are metabolic products and
    inhibit cellular metabolism
    C. there may be a delay in onset of symptoms of from sev-
    eral hours to two days
    D. gastric lavage is of no value because of rapidity of ab-
    sorption from the stomach
    E. optic atrophy may follow recovery from acute poisoning

177. A diagnosis of atropine poisoning may be confused with
    A. scarlet fever
    B. chickenpox
    C. cholera
    D. vitamin C deficiency
    E. acute appendicitis

178. Which of the following is associated with hemolysis of red
blood cells resulting in hemoglobinuria and hematuria?
    A. Barium salts
    B. Naphthalene
    C. Atropine
    D. Carbon monoxide
    E. Cyanide

179. A two-year-old had ingested an Indan derivative (chlordane). The calculated ingestion is 0.5 gm/kg. The cause of death is most likely to be a result of
   A. gastrointestinal tract perforation and bleeding
   B. clotting problem and hemolysis
   C. hematuria and oliguria
   D. liver failure
   E. central nervous system depression with respiratory failure

180. All of the following statements regarding iron (ferrous salt) toxicity are correct EXCEPT
   A. oral ingestion of 2 to 4 gm of soluble iron salts may be fatal in 50% of cases
   B. hemodynamic changes produce shock and CNS depression
   C. early symptoms are a result of GI tract irritation
   D. direct hepatic damage may occur
   E. alkalosis occurs and is corrected with acids

181. A four-year-old has been taken to an emergency room because of accidental poisoning with phenobarbital. The child should be treated with
   A. N-allylnormorphine (Nalline)
   B. L-3 hydroxy-N-allylmorphinan tartrate (Lorfan)
   C. naloxone (Narcan)
   D. epinephrine
   E. none of the above

182. All of the following statements regarding acrodynia are correct EXCEPT
   A. acrodynia is the result of chronic mercury poisoning
   B. the natural course is prolonged from several months to a year
   C. in the early course the tips of the fingers, toes, and nose acquire a pinkish color. Later on, the hands and feet become a dusky pink with areas of ischemia
   D. prolapse of the rectum is a frequent complication
   E. pathognomonic changes in the CSF include increased protein, decreased sugar, and 20 to 30 mononuclear cells

183. The chronic encephalopathy of lead poisoning includes all of the following EXCEPT
   A. seizure disorders, hyperkinetic and aggressive behavior disorders
   B. developmental regression and progressive loss of speech
   C. lack of evidence of acutely increased intracranial pressure
   D. initial symptom is peripheral neuropathy
   E. attentional deficit disorder due to subclinical lead poisoning

---

DIRECTIONS: This section consists of situations, each followed by a series of questions. Study each situation, and select the **one** best answer to each question following it.

CASE 1 (Questions 184–186): A four-year-old girl has been playing with her mother's necklace. She is found with the string broken and the ornamental beans scattered and is suspected of accidental ingestion. She is brought to the emergency room with the beans of the necklace; they are scarlet with a black core at the hilus.

184. The description of the bean resembles that of the
   A. castor bean
   B. jequirity bean
   C. holly bean
   D. baked bean
   E. lima bean

185. In the emergency room, the physician should not be concerned because
   A. the bean is nontoxic
   B. the bean must be consumed in large quantities to be considered toxic
   C. the child probably did not chew a bean
   D. the bean only caused diarrhea
   E. none of the above

186. The major pathology caused by poisoning with the bean is
   A. CNS stimulation
   B. CNS depression
   C. hemolysis
   D. oil pneumonia
   E. gastric ulceration and perforation

CASE 2 (Questions 187-188): A two-year-old boy is brought to your office because of "headache and dizziness." Examination reveals shallow respirations, cyanosis, and hypotension. A rash believed to be an allergy is found in the elbow creases. An x-ray of the abdomen reveals small opaque fragments. The child's mother reports he was playing with a coloring book and some old wax crayons prior to "getting sick." In the child's room she found some fragments of leaves from a household plant, but, she believes the dog chewed on them.

187. From the description, the most likely possibility is
   A. lead intoxication
   B. rare plant intoxication
   C. botulism
   D. paranitraniline intoxication
   E. mercury poisoning

188. Treatment should include all of the following EXCEPT
   A. repeated gastric lavage
   B. lavage followed by catharsis
   C. oxygen
   D. transfusion, exchange transfusion, and methylene blue
   E. topical antibiotics for the elbow rash

CASE 3 (Questions 189-190): A five-day-old infant is being treated by grandmother for "severe diaper rash." Home remedy consists of boric acid soaks to the area and thick boric acid paste to the open lesions. The child is seen by a physician and meningeal signs are noted. The infant is hospitalized and a convulsion is noted on admission. After appropriate CNS studies, a diagnosis of boric acid toxicity is considered.

189. Boric acid toxicity is associated with all of the following EXCEPT
   A. it may result from application as a wet dressing or as an ointment
   B. mortality in infants is about 70%
   C. excretion of boric acid is slow; a cumulative action may result
   D. a rash confined to the trunk is observed
   E. in infants signs of meningeal irritation may occur

190. Treatment for boric acid toxicity in this case is
   A. BAL intramuscularly
   B. supportive care with oxygen and fluids
   C. methylene blue
   D. intravenous ephedrine, followed by diazepam
   E. none of the above

IV: Accidents, Poisonings, and Environmental Hazards
Answers and Comments

153. E. Accident-proneness is a controversial issue. It does not eliminate the need for adult supervision of the dangerous environment. Indeed, it demands more adult concern for such a child's environment. Virtually all accidents are preventable. The hyperactive, impulsive, short-attentioned, emotionally labile child may be more prone to accidents but needs tighter supervision as a preventative measure. *(REF. 1 — p. 765)*

154. D. Consciousness and absence of apnea in drowning victims are *not* reliable signs of assured recovery. Lethal secondary drowning can occur after rescue. Lethal secondary drowning is an especial danger following seawater drowning. Hospitalization for observation is recommended. *(REF. 1 — pp. 766–768)*

155. C. Spilling a hot liquid onto himself and immersion in scalding liquids represent the most common etiology for burns in childhood. Scald burns are less likely to be fatal than immersion scald burns because of the differences in surface area involved. *(REF. 1 — pp. 770, 771)*

156. A. The use of hexachlorophene is contraindicated because surface absorption may result in neurotoxicity. Topical antibiotics are not utilized for out-patient care. Superficial burns such as this are not tetanus-prone. Routine oral antibiotics are not necessary. *(REF. 1 — pp. 772–773)*

157. A. Drugs that are poorly secured are the most common causes of childhood poisonings. The involved agents are aspirin, hematinics, vitamins, antihistamines, tranquilizers, analgesics, and cough medicines. *(REF. 1 — p. 780)*

158. D. From the list one would think first of the castor bean because of the characteristic features described. The poisonous substance of the castor bean is ricin. Larkspur causes CNS excitation; oleander, CNS depression, bradyarrhythmia; jimsonweed has an atropine-like effect; and azalea has a curare-like effect. *(REF. 1 — p. 781)*

159. B. Gastric lavage would be indicated for all of the accidental ingestions except corrosive agents. The risk involves possible perforation of the esophagus. Children with strychnine, glutethimide, barbiturate, or antihistamine poisoning may require prior endotracheal intubation because of the danger of laryngospasm. *(REF. 1 — p. 783)*

160. C. Toxic levels of salicylate produce an encephalopathy with primary disturbance of the respiratory center of the medulla, resulting in a primary hyperpnea. A result of the primary hyperventilation is reduced PCO_2, which causes a rise in plasma pH. *(REF. 1 — p. 788)*

161. A. The first phase of iron toxicity usually begins within 30 to 60 minutes after ingestion. Usually, the initial signs are vomiting and bloody diarrhea; acidemia and circulatory collapse may develop. *(REF. 1 — p. 791)*

162. A. Aspiration of hydrocarbon into the respiratory tract causes local irritation pneumonitis, hemorrhagic bronchopneumonia, atelectasis, and pulmonary edema. Complications include pneumatoceles, effusions and pneumothorax. Extensive lesions in the lungs can cause death within two to 24 hours after ingestion. *(REF. 1 — p. 796)*

163. B. All effects described are correct, except there is a lowering of body temperature. The heroin appears to exert a direct effect on the hypothalamus. *(REF. 1 — pp. 809–810)*

164. B. Until proved otherwise, the patient must be considered to have overdosed on heroin. Methadone overdose is identical to that of heroin. Toxicity from barbiturates also resembles that from opiates. *(REF. 1 — p. 813)*

165. E. Alcohol is the most commonly abused agent. Teenagers use and experiment with alcohol, more so than with tobacco or marijuana. It is estimated that there are 500,000 teenage alcoholics. *(REF. 1 — p. 822)*

166. A. The incidence of drowning is highest among the 10-19 year age group. *(REF. 2 — p. 319)*

167. B. Ten percent of victims die of laryngospasm or breath-holding. With prompt resuscitation recovery is complete. *(REF. 2 — p. 319)*

168. C. In the U.S. over 7,000 deaths due to drowning are recorded annually. *(REF. 2 — p. 319)*

169. A. In botulism, the CNS symptoms usually develop within 12 to 48 hours. The signs are a result of a curare-like action of the toxin on the motor end plate. *(REF. 2 — pp. 809–810)*

170. A. Causative exotoxins have been demonstrated for *Clostridium botulinum* and *Staphylococcus aureus*. *(REF. 2 — p. 753)*

171. A. Accidents and poisonings account for more than the next seven causes of death combined. They rank first as the most common pediatric emergency. More than 3,000 fatal poisonings occur each year in persons of all ages; four-fifths are in children 4 years of age. *(REF. 3 — p. 1660)*

172. D. In this age group the five most common causes of poisoning include (in order of frequency) aspirin, soaps, detergents, cleansers, and bleaches. Poisoning is more frequent in boys than in girls less than five years of age. *(REF. 3 — p. 1660)*

173. C. All of the agents cited produce dilated pupils except for muscarine which causes pinpoint pupils. *(REF. 3 — p. 1661)*

174. E. The agents in A, B, C, & D commonly produce methemoglobinemia, which causes anoxia and convulsions. Chloral hydrate causes anoxia and produces coma, but does not do so by methemoglobinemia formation. *(REF. 3 — p. 1661)*

175. E. Extreme caution is required with this child. Lavage may cause enough stimulation to produce a fatal convulsion. Lavage with 2% tannic acid or strong tea binds the alkaloid. *(REF. 3 — p. 1662)*

176. D. All of the facts stated except D relate to methyl alcohol poisoning. Treatment includes gastric lavage, repeated over several days; intravenous alkali to combat severe acidosis; and potassium for hypokalemia. Peritoneal dialysis can reduce the blood level of methanol. Gastric lavage may be repeated over 24 to 48 hours because methanol may be resecreted into the stomach. *(REF. 3 — p. 1665)*

177. A. In atropine poisoning, there may be confusion with scarlet fever because the onset of the latter may be associated with rash, fever, tachycardia, and delirium. *(REF. 3 — p. 1666)*

178. B. Naphthalene, a benzene derivative, is the common ingredient of moth repellents. The compound causes hemolysis of red blood cells. Hemoglobinuria and hematuria can result from hemolysis. Blood transfusions and exchange transfusions may be of value. *(REF. 3 — pp. 1666–1669)*

179. E. The usual cause of death with chlordane poisoning is central nervous system depression with respiratory failure. Recovery is more likely if convulsions are delayed or prevented. Convulsions may be controlled with barbiturates. Stimulants are to be avoided. and epinephrine is contraindicated. *(REF. 3 — p. 1668)*

180. E. All of the statements are correct, except for E. In this poisoning, acidosis occurs as a result of the accumulation of lactic and citric acids. The organic acidosis is treated with sodium bicarbonate. *(REF. 2 — p. 2019)*

181. E. All three drugs have specific antagonistic actions against all opiates. They are ineffective against phenobarbital. Nalline and Lorfan will produce toxic effects of opiates if used for poisoning other than opiate poisoning. *(REF. 2 — pp. 2017–2018)*

182. E. There are no pathognomonic signs in the blood, urine, or CSF. There are no characteristic changes in the spinal fluid. There may be some proteinuria. Laboratory data are of little value except for demonstrating the presence of mercury. *(REF. 2 — pp. 2023–2024)*

183. D. All of the statements except D are correct and may occur as a result of acute encephalopathy or chronic ingestion of lead. Sequelae include seizure disorders, hyperkinesis, and intellectual deficits. Subclinical lead intoxication has been implicated in attentional deficit disorder. It may be associated with impaired learning and hyperkinesis. Peripheral neuropathy as a complication of plumbism is rare in children. It is observed in adults as motor weakness in the distal muscles and in the arms and legs. *(REF. 2 — p. 2027)*

184. B. The description fits that of the jequirity bean. It is commonly used for necklaces, bead bags, moccasins, rosaries, earrings, etc. *(REF. 3 — p. 1664)*

185. E. There should be concern, for one bean thoroughly chewed can be fatal. The treatment should include gastric lavage, catharsis, and supportive treatment. *(REF. 3 — p. 1665)*

186. C. Jequirity beans (*Abrus precatorius*) cause hemolysis of red blood cells in extreme dilutions. *(REF. 3 — p. 1665)*

187. D. The clinical symptoms suggest poisoning within the group of agents: aniline, dimethylaniline nitroaniline, nitrobenzene, acetophenetidin, etc. The crayons (and x-ray evidence of ingestion) may have contained paranitraniline. They are more often found in yellow and orange wax crayons. *(REF. 3 — p. 1665)*

188. E. All of the measures suggested may be necessary. The symptoms as described may progress to include convulsions and coma. However, topical antibiotics are not indicated for the associated rash. The rash will not respond to this regimen for obvious reasons. *(REF. 3 — p. 1665)*

189. D. All of the statements are true concerning boric acid toxicity except D. In infants, signs of meningeal irritation may occur, followed by convulsion, delirium, and coma. Albuminuria and azotemia may develop. The rash of boric acid toxicity has been described as maculopapular, urticarial, or scarlatiniform. It can be observed on the palms and soles. Desquamation may occur in several days. *(REF. 3 — p. 1667)*

190. E. Although treatment is symptomatic in this case because of the CNS problems, exchange transfusion or hemodialysis may be lifesaving. *(REF. 3 — p. 1667)*

V: Nutrition

191. The LEAST digestible source(s) of nitrogen in the human diet is(are)
    A. milk and milk products
    B. eggs
    C. animal muscle protein
    D. vegetable protein
    E. fish protein

192. Amino acids in excess of needs for protein synthesis and other nitrogen compounds are handled in all of the following ways EXCEPT
    A. excreted as ammonia
    B. stored as amino acids in the liver
    C. synthesized into energy-yielding compounds
    D. synthesized into storage compounds such as fat
    E. excreted as urea

193. Essential amino acids for the neonate which are the same as for the older child include all of the following EXCEPT
    A. valine
    B. lysine
    C. leucine
    D. phenylalanine
    E. cystine

194. For which of the following reasons are basal metabolism rates of children higher than those of adults?
    A. Hormonal activity differences
    B. Less efficient gastrointestinal absorption of nutrients
    C. Growth and greater heat loss per unit of weight
    D. Children are more physically active
    E. Higher metabolic rate of the liver

195. The essential fatty acid(s) required in small amounts in the diet is(are)
    A. none, because the human can synthesize all fatty acids from carbohydrates and protein intake
    B. cholesterol and linoleic acid
    C. linoleic and arachidonic acids
    D. linoleic acid (which is the only true essential fatty acid)
    E. all of the polyunsaturated fats

196. In comparing the lipid content of human milk with that of modified cow-milk formula, all of the following are true EXCEPT
    A. the cholesterol content of human milk is highest
    B. the lipid composition of human milk contains more saturated fatty acids
    C. human milk is higher in essential fatty acids
    D. avoidance of human milk for infant feeding is a proved preventive measure for atheromatous disease in later life
    E. human milk fat is easily absorbed by the infant

197. Fat depot in individuals of normal body weight constitutes what percentage of body weight?
    A. 20%
    B. 25%
    C. 2%
    D. 35%
    E. 10%

198. Patients at risk for pernicious anemia include all of the following EXCEPT
    A. vegetarians who include eggs and milk
    B. postgastrectomy patients
    C. patients with ileal resection
    D. patients lacking intrinsic factor for B_{12} absorption
    E. vegetarians who consume large amounts of nut proteins

199. Which of the following statements concerning vitamin K is FALSE?
- **A.** Its major source is dietary fat
- **B.** Deficiency in newborn may result in bleeding
- **C.** Production by intestinal bacteria ordinarily meets the requirement
- **D.** Prolonged administration of antibiotics may effect vitamin levels
- **E.** Deficiency in newborn may not result in bleeding

200. A 15-year-old male places himself on a protein-sparing fast. His diet consists only of raw egg white. All of the following would be expected to occur EXCEPT
- **A.** weight loss
- **B.** ketosis
- **C.** dermatitis
- **D.** an excess of the vitamin biotin in body tissues
- **E.** decrease of the vitamin biotin in body tissues

201. All of the following statements concerning vitamin E are true EXCEPT
- **A.** premature infants and cystic fibrosis patients are at risk for vitamin E deficiency as demonstrated by a positive RBC hydrogen peroxide test
- **B.** vitamin E is an effective antioxidant
- **C.** serum $\alpha2$-tocopherol levels are not yet available.
- **D.** large amounts of polyunsaturated fat in the diet may require increased amount of vitamin E
- **E.** vitamin E is considered a relatively safe vitamin when consumed in amounts above the RDA

202. Colostrum has all of the following properties EXCEPT
- **A.** it has higher fat content than mature milk
- **B.** it has higher protein content than mature milk
- **C.** it is richer in vitamin A as compared to mature human milk
- **D.** sodium and potassium are higher than in mature human milk
- **E.** it contains protective antibodies

203. Which of the following statements is true of antigenic substances in breast milk?
   A. May prove to be a valid reason for weaning
   B. Frequently proved as a cause of allergic reactions in the infant
   C. Allergic reaction is always manifested in part by oral dermatitis
   D. Possible problems can be avoided by administration of oral antihistamine to the infant
   E. Allergic reaction is always in the form of vomiting

204. An absolute contraindication to breast feeding is
   A. erythroblastosis fetalis
   B. inverted nipples
   C. mastitis
   D. cigarette smoking
   E. active tuberculosis in the mother

205. All of the following apply to a comparison between breast milk and cow's milk EXCEPT
   A. breast milk produces lower stool pH
   B. breast milk produces higher counts of lactobacillus in stools
   C. breast milk produces high concentrations of secretory IgA
   D. breast milk has a lower caloric content
   E. fat absorption by infant is better with breast milk

206. Regarding routine immunizations in breast-fed infants, which of the following approaches should be employed?
   A. Breast milk should be withheld for 12 hours before any immunization is given
   B. Consumption of breast milk within two hours of oral polio vaccine will render the immunization completely ineffective
   C. The feeding of breast milk and oral polio vaccine administration produces mild diarrhea in the majority of infants and requires the use of antidiarrheal drugs
   D. Breast-fed infants should not receive polio immunization
   E. Breast-fed infants can be safely and effectively immunized with both DPT and oral polio vaccine

207. For the very small premature infant, breast milk may provide inadequate amounts of
    A. calories
    B. fat
    C. lactose
    D. calcium
    E. vitamin C

208. A mother should be advised of which of the following if she decides to breast-feed for six months?
    A. Her breast will be reduced in size permanently
    B. Her breast will be increased in size permanently
    C. Probably no change from pre-pregnancy breast size will occur
    D. The results as to change in breast size are so unpredictable
    E. None of the above, since mothers who desire to breast-feed are unconcerned about the subject of breast size postlactation

209. Electric breast pumps are
    A. useful in the management of engorged breasts
    B. unavailable in this country
    C. conducive to permanent breast damage
    D. contraindicated because of the high risk of infection
    E. effective but cause moderate pain to the user

210. Which of the following is an absolute contraindication to breast-feeding in the first month of life?
    A. Prematurity of the infant
    B. Sickle cell disease in the mother
    C. Fe-deficiency anemia in the mother
    D. Unsupportive father
    E. Sulfonamide drug therapy of maternal infection

211. All of the following observations might be indicators of the adequacy of breast milk supply EXCEPT
    A. if the infant appears satisfied
    B. if the infant sleeps two to four hours between feedings
    C. if the infant exhibits adequate weight gain
    D. if the mother has a let-down reflex and feels breasts are emptied after feedings
    E. if the infant rarely cries

212. Which of the following infant feedings provides 3 to 4 gm/kg/day of protein?
    A. Breast milk
    B. Soy protein formula
    C. Evaporated cow's milk at 1:1 dilution
    D. Commercial modified cow milk infant formula
    E. Evaporated cow's milk at 1:2 dilution

213. An infant feeding composed of 60% whey proteins and 40% casein is
    A. evaporated cow's milk at 1:1 dilution
    B. whole cow's milk
    C. breast milk
    D. skim cow's milk
    E. goat's milk

214. Concerning colostrum, which of the following statements is FALSE?
    A. It has an alkaline reaction
    B. It secretes 10 to 40 ml daily
    C. It contains less protein than breast milk
    D. It contains less carbohydrate and fat than breast milk
    E. It contains maternal leukocytes

215. Hypoallergenic infant milks include all of the following EX-CEPT
    A. goat milk formulas
    B. casein hydrolysate formula
    C. human milk
    D. soy formulas
    E. modified cow milk formula

216. By seven months of age most infants have adjusted to a feeding schedule of
    A. 2 times a day
    B. 6 times a day
    C. 4 times a day
    D. 3 times a day
    E. 8 times a day

217. How many calories per day does a one-month-old infant weighing 5 kg require for adequate growth?
    A. 900–1,100
    B. 700–900
    C. 200–300
    D. 150–200
    E. 500–600

218. Introduction of semisolid feeding to infants less than two months of age may result in all of the following EXCEPT
    A. infantile obesity
    B. unbalanced diet
    C. the infant may resist swallowing by reflex mechanisms
    D. decreased formula intake
    E. intestinal obstruction

219. Protein malnutrition during infancy may result in all of the following EXCEPT
    A. dermatitis
    B. red-haired black children
    C. edema
    D. increased serum proteins
    E. low-serum albumin

220. The caloric-excess obese child as compared to his normal-weight cohort may
    A. have decreased bone age
    B. be shorter
    C. show a high incidence of micropenis
    D. have advanced bone age
    E. have decreased muscle mass

221. The most frequent time for the appearance of obesity in childhood is the
    A. first year of life
    B. third year of life
    C. ninth year of life
    D. eighth year of life
    E. tenth year of life

222. The presence of unusual amounts of carotene in the blood may be associated with all of the following EXCEPT
    A. yellow discoloration of the scleras
    B. hypothyroidism
    C. liver disease
    D. congenital absence of enzymes necessary to convert pro-vitamin A carotenoids
    E. large amounts of carotene-containing foods in the diet, such as carrots

223. Vitamin A deficiency can be expected to occur with all of the following EXCEPT
    A. chronic ingestion of mineral oil
    B. a low-fat diet
    C. pancreatic disease
    D. celiac disease
    E. a lack of yellow vegetables in the diet

224. Hypervitaminosis A may be associated with all of the following EXCEPT
    A. acute ingestion of 300,000 IU of vitamin A
    B. symptoms of pseudotumor cerebri
    C. anorexia and vomiting
    D. blood levels of retinol in the range of 20 to 50 μg/dl
    E. desquamation of the skin

225. The breast-fed infant of a mother with severe beriberi would be expected to exhibit all of the following EXCEPT
    A. restlessness, anorexia, vomiting, and constipation
    B. undernourishment
    C. rapid heart rate and enlarged liver
    D. edema restricted to the head and trunk
    E. waxy skin

226. Niacin deficiency is characterized by
    A. an increased incidence in patients on vegetarian diets with milk and eggs included
    B. diarrhea, dermatitis, and dementia
    C. a dermatitis that responds to exposure to sunlight
    D. an increased incidence in fall and winter
    E. high morbidity

227. Pyridoxine deficiency may be associated with all of the following EXCEPT
    A. seizure disorder
    B. isoniazid ingestion
    C. a macrocytic anemia
    D. ingestion of prolonged heat-processed formula by infants
    E. inherited inability to utilize normal amounts of pyridoxine

228. The need for vitamin C is increased by all of the following EXCEPT
    A. infectious disease
    B. iron deficiency
    C. smoking
    D. cold exposure
    E. protein excess in diet

229. Approximately how many mg/dl of ascorbic acid does breast milk contain?
    A. 20 to 30
    B. 1 to 2
    C. 4 to 7
    D. 50 to 100
    E. 100 to 200

230. The vitamin C content of cord blood plasma is how many times greater than maternal plasma?
    A. 10 to 20
    B. 6 to 8
    C. 2 to 4
    D. 50 to 75
    E. 30 to 40

231. Defects in the formation of which of the following explain most of the clinical findings in scurvy?
    A. Phospholipid
    B. Protein
    C. Endothelium
    D. Glycogen
    E. Collagen

232. Scurvy is a manifestation of a deficiency of which of the following?
    A. Vitamin C
    B. Vitamin B
    C. Vitamin K
    D. Vitamin E
    E. Vitamin A

233. A ten-month-old infant with known iron deficiency, fed solely on cow's milk, develops painful lower extremities, refuses to walk, and assumes a "frog position" when resting. The most likely nutritional disorder is
    A. protein-calorie malnutrition
    B. scurvy
    C. vitamin D rickets
    D. B-complex deficiency
    E. vitamin A deficiency

234. Anemia may result in vitamin C deficiency because of
    A. hemolysis
    B. impaired Fe utilization
    C. massive GI bleeding
    D. maturation arrest of RBC
    E. increased need for collagen formation

235. The diagnosis of scurvy is usually made by
    A. blood assay
    B. tissue biopsy
    C. x-ray of long bones
    D. assay of nail content
    E. radioactive isotope methods

236. For infants, the daily intake of vitamin C should be
    A. 150 mg
    B. 200 mg
    C. 25 to 50 mg
    D. 75 to 100 mg
    E. 100 to 250 mg

237. The vitamin deficiency that produces osteomalacia in non-growing bone is
   A. vitamin C
   B. vitamin A
   C. vitamin B_6
   D. vitamin B_2
   E. vitamin D

238. The skin contains 7-dehydrocholesterol. This provitamin D_3 will be activated by
   A. exposure to outdoor sunlight
   B. exposure to sun through window glass
   C. exposure to cold
   D. rubbing the skin
   E. none of the above

239. Which of the following statements concerning vitamin D metabolism is FALSE?
   A. Bound to alpha-2 globin in lymphatics
   B. Requires bile for absorption
   C. Kidney is active in metabolism
   D. Circulates in plasma as 25-OH cholecalciferol
   E. Stored in the liver but is not metabolized there

240. In the absence of vitamin D, serum calcium may be maintained by
   A. parathyroid hormone secretion
   B. decreased renal excretion of phosphate
   C. small dietary increases
   D. decreased renal excretion of alkali
   E. increased amounts of vitamin A in diet

241. Clinical disorders associated with increased incidence of vitamin D deficiency include all of the following EXCEPT
   A. cystic fibrosis
   B. hepatic disease
   C. celiac disease
   D. renal disease
   E. obesity

242. With treatment the bony changes of rickets may experience total repair
    A. within one week of vitamin D administration
    B. within months or years
    C. never in the majority of cases
    D. within two days of vitamin D administration
    E. only if high-dose calcium supplementation is also used

243. A frayed irregular epiphyseal line at the end of the shaft of the femur may be seen in a deficiency of vitamin
    A. B_6
    B. C
    C. D
    D. A
    E. E

244. Maximum calcium absorption occurs in children when the ratio of calcium to phosphorus in the diet is about
    A. 2:1
    B. 4:1
    C. 1:1
    D. 1:2
    E. 1:4

245. All of the following are effects of parathyroid hormone EXCEPT
    A. hypophosphatemia
    B. hyperphosphaturia
    C. calcium release from bone
    D. reduced renal clearance of calcium
    E. decreased calcium absorption from gut

246. Which of the following statements concerning calcitonin is FALSE?
    A. It is secreted by the kidney
    B. It inhibits bone resorption
    C. It lowers serum calcium in hypercalcemia
    D. The activity of calcitonin increases with increasing levels of serum phosphate
    E. A thyroidectomy causes decreased secretion of calcitonin

247. All of the following are clinical signs of rickets EXCEPT
    A. craniotabes
    B. enlargement of costochondral junctions
    C. thickening of wrists and ankles
    D. poor growth
    E. conjunctivitis

248. Harrison's groove, caput quadratum, and pigeon breast deformity would probably all be found in an infant with a deficiency of
    A. vitamin C
    B. vitamin D
    C. magnesium
    D. calcium
    E. vitamin A

249. The x-ray that will help diagnose rickets early is one of the
    A. lumbar spine
    B. chest with rib detail
    C. wrist
    D. hip
    E. elbow

250. The daily requirement for vitamin D is
    A. 100 IU
    B. 400 IU
    C. 600 IU
    D. 1,000 IU
    E. 50 IU

251. Rickets may be treated by all of the following EXCEPT
    A. sunlight
    B. 1,500 to 5,000 IU of vitamin D daily for two to four weeks
    C. 600,000 IU of vitamin D as a single dose
    D. sunlight plus 1,500 to 5,000 IU of vitamin D daily until healing is demonstrated on x-ray
    E. increased calcium in diet and decreased phosphate

252. Symptoms of hypervitaminosis D include all of the following EXCEPT
   A. hypotonia
   B. polydipsia and polyuria
   C. irritability
   D. hypocalcemia
   E. metastatic calcifications

253. Vitamin E deficiency may develop with all of the following EXCEPT
   A. prematures
   B. cystic fibrosis
   C. kwashiorkor
   D. dietary intake of 1 mg of vitamin E per 0.6 gm of unsaturated fat in diet
   E. biliary atresia

254. Children receiving large doses of salicylates may require additional amounts of
   A. vitamin D
   B. vitamin K
   C. vitamin C
   D. vitamin A
   E. vitamin E

255. Which of the following statements is FALSE concerning the effects of rickets on the teeth of infants?
   A. Delayed eruption
   B. Eruption order is abnormal
   C. Caries in deciduous teeth
   D. Permanent teeth are affected
   E. Dental defects are very rare

256. Which of the following statements concerning body water is FALSE?
   A. TBW decreases from 78% of body weight at birth to 60% at one year of age
   B. Extracellular fluid volume is larger than intracellular space in the fetus
   C. Extracellular fluid volume is approximately 40% of body weight in the older child
   D. Intracellular fluid volume is approximately 30% to 40% of body weight
   E. TBW (liters) = 0.611 wt (kg) ± 0.251

257. Intracellular fluid volume is approximately what percent of body weight in the child older than 1 year?
   A. 30 to 40
   B. 10 to 20
   C. 50 to 60
   D. 60 to 70
   E. 70 to 80

258. The principal regulatory mechanism for water excretion is
   A. glomerular filtration rate
   B. the adrenal gland
   C. antidiuretic hormone
   D. the state of the renal tubular epithelium
   E. the sweat gland

259. Release of ADH may be stimulated by all of the following EXCEPT
   A. decrease in effective arterial blood volume
   B. nicotine
   C. pain
   D. hypertonic saline
   E. urea

260. The largest concentration of sodium in the body is in
   A. bone
   B. plasma
   C. interstitial fluid
   D. intracellular fluid
   E. liver

261. Which of the following statements concerning sodium regulation is FALSE?
   A. Infants have a relatively high sodium intake
   B. The regulatory mechanism for sodium intake is poorly developed
   C. The sodium content of the fetus is relatively higher than that of the adult
   D. Absorption of sodium occurs only in the distal ileum
   E. Patients with cystic fibrosis are prone to hyponatremia

262. Which of the following statements concerning body potassium is FALSE?
    A. Ninety-five percent is exchangeable
    B. Bulk is intracellular
    C. Total body potassium is highly correlated with body weight and height
    D. Most intracellular potassium is bound
    E. Extracellular concentration is 4 to 5 mEq/L

263. Total body sodium is depleted in all of the following EXCEPT
    A. hyponatremic dehydration
    B. isonatremic dehydration
    C. hypernatremic dehydration
    D. Addison's disease
    E. Cushing's disease

264. Which is the appropriate IV fluid for initial hydration of the patient with severe hypernatremic dehydration?
    A. Five percent glucose in water
    B. Isotonic saline with potassium
    C. Ten percent glucose in water
    D. Sodium in glucose solution without potassium
    E. Two and one-half percent glucose in water

265. Improvement in a hospitalized infant who had failed to gain weight and was developmentally slow at home would suggest
    A. an infectious etiology
    B. carbon monoxide poisoning
    C. psychosocial factors
    D. rumination syndrome
    E. food intolerance

V: Nutrition
Answers and Comments

191. D. Probably because of fiber content but possibly also because of molecular structure, the proteins of vegetable origin are considered the least digestible. *(REF. 1 — p. 187)*

192. B. There is no storage facility for amino acids. *(REF. 1 — p. 187)*

193. E. Fetuses, small premature infants, and possibly some full-term infants may have a very limited capacity to convert methionine to cysteine and cystine. *(REF. 1 — p. 190)*

194. C. Basal metabolism rates of children are higher than those of adults because of growth and greater heat loss per unit of weight. *(REF. 1 — p. 187)*

195. D. Linoleic acid has been conclusively proved to be an essential nutrient for both children and adults. Arachidonic acid performs some of the same functions, but it is not essential because it can be synthesized from linoleic acid. *(REF. 1 — p. 193)*

196. D. Avoidance of the higher cholesterol content of human milk has not been proved to modify atheromatous disease of later life. It is an area under investigation. *(REF. 1 — p. 193)*

197. E. The normal is 10%. In extreme obesity the depot may exceed 50%. In states of starvation, less than 1% of total body weight may be devoted to fat. *(REF. 1 — p. 193)*

198. A. B_{12} is present in sufficient amounts in egg and milk products and will protect the patient who has excluded meat from his diet. *(REF. 1 — p. 195)*

199. A. The major source of vitamin K is synthesis by intestinal bacteria. It is present in some natural fats. *(REF. 1 — p. 196)*

200. D. A deficiency of biotin results when liberal amounts of raw egg white are included in the diet. The egg white protein avidin inactivates biotin, which is synthesized by intestinal bacteria. *(REF. 1 — p. 196)*

201. C. Serum and tissue vitamin E levels are available. *(REF. 1 — pp. 196–197)*

202. A. Colostrum has less fat and sugar than mature milk. *(REF. 1 — p. 203)*

203. A. Allergens to which the infant is sensitized are infrequently carried in breast milk, but on rare occasions the possibility of such is entertained when the symptoms disappear with weaning. Allergic symptoms may vary widely depending upon the organ system affected. *(REF. 2 — p. 192)*

204. E. Active tuberculosis is an absolute contraindication as are other serious maternal infections. *(REF. 2 — p. 192)*

205. D. Total caloric content is the same, but caloric distribution is significantly different. *(REF. 2 — pp. 191, 197–199)*

206. E. Breast-fed infants can be immunized safely and effectively with oral polio vaccine with no need to withhold feedings. Any symptoms from the routine immunizations are the same as might be seen in a non-breast-fed infant. *(REF. 2 — p. 192)*

207. D. Calcium may be proved to be inadequate for normal growth in infants less than 1,500 grams. *(REF. 2 — p. 192)*

208. C. With proper support during the nursing period, few mothers will have significant change in breast size. *(REF. 2 — p. 193)*

209. A. Breast pumps are readily available in the U.S. and are a safe and useful apparatus for emptying the breasts. *(REF. 2 — pp. 193, 196)*

210. E. Sulfonamides are excreted in breast milk and are a contraindication to breast-feeding in the first few weeks of life because of their effects on bilirubin binding. *(REF. 2 — p. 194)*

211. E. Infants cry for many reasons other than hunger. Usually the best single indicator of adequate breast milk supply is growth of the infant. *(REF. 2 — p. 195)*

212. C. Evaporated cow's milk formula at 1:1 dilution provides infants with a relatively large protein excess. All of the other infant feedings listed provide 1 to 2.5 gm/kg/body weight of protein. *(REF. 2 — p. 197)*

213. C. Cow's milk protein's whey/casein ratio is 18:82. *(REF. 2 — p. 198)*

214. C. Colostrum contains several times as much protein as breast milk. *(REF. 2 — p. 198)*

215. E. All the formulas listed, except modified cow milk, may prove to be of use in the infant with cow-milk allergy. *(REF. 2 — p. 201)*

216. C. Usual adjustment is four to five feedings a day. *(REF. 2 — p. 205)*

217. E. Five-hundred to 600 cal/day would supply the infant with 100 to 120 cal/kg/day. *(REF. 2 — p. 201)*

218. E. There is no nutritional necessity for introduction of this type of feeding at two months of age, but intestinal obstruction has not been observed. Constipation may result and diarrhea is not an uncommon occurrence. *(REF. 2 — p. 206)*

219. D. Serum proteins may be normal or serum albumin may be reduced. *(REF. 2 — pp. 213-214)*

220. D. Bone age and height may be increased for chronological age in the caloric-excess obese child. *(REF. 2 — p. 216)*

221. A. The first year of life, at five to six years of age, and adolescence are the most frequent times for the onset of obesity. *(REF. 2 — p. 216)*

222. A. Carotenemia produces yellow discoloration of skin, but the scleras remain unaffected. *(REF. 2 — p. 217)*

223. E. All of the choices presented except the lack of yellow vegetables in the diet can result in low intake of or poor absorption of vitamin A. Fruits, eggs, butter, and liver provide adequate amounts of vitamin A. *(REF. 2 — pp. 218-219)*

224. D. Blood levels of retinol in the range of 20 to 50 μg/dl are normal for infants. *(REF. 2 — p. 219)*

225. D. Congenital beriberi has been described in breast-fed infants of mothers with severe beriberi. They usually become symptomatic during the first three months of life. The edema, if present, is usually restricted to the distal parts of the extremities. *(REF. 2 — p. 221)*

226. B. The classic triad of pellagra consists of diarrhea, dermatitis, and dementia. *(REF. 2 — p. 222)*

227. C. The anemia of pyridoxine deficiency is a microcytic hypochromic anemia associated with failure of iron utilization in hemoglobin synthesis. *(REF. 2 — p. 224)*

228. E. Protein depletion may increase the need for vitamin C. *(REF. 2 — p. 225)*

229. C. Breast milk contains 4 to 7 mg/dl and is an adequate source of vitamin C for the infant. *(REF. 2 — p. 225)*

230. C. Cord blood will have two to four times as much vitamin C. *(REF. 2 — p. 225)*

231. E. Ascorbate and oxygen are essential for formation of normal collagen. *(REF. 2 — p. 225)*

232. A. Vitamin C deficiency will result in a symptom complex called scurvy. *(REF. 2 — p. 225)*

233. B. A diet consisting solely of cow's milk would be deficient in vitamin C. The pain-associated periosteal lesions cause pseudoparalysis. *(REF. 2 — pp. 225–226)*

234. B. Impaired folic acid metabolism may also result in anemia. *(REF. 2 — pp. 225–227)*

235. C. Laboratory tests for scurvy are unsatisfactory. The characteristic clinical picture and history are valuable in diagnosis. *(REF. 2 — p. 226)*

236. C. Twenty-five to 50 mg of ascorbic acid is the recommendation for infants; for the older child, 50 mg. *(REF. 2 — p. 228)*

237. E. Rickets (vitamin D deficiency) is characterized by formation of normal collagen and matrix and of osteoid, with defective mineralization. *(REF. 2 — p. 228)*

238. A. Provitamin D_3 is activated by sunlight. Ordinary window glass will prevent this process. *(REF. 2 — p. 228)*

239. E. Vitamin D_3 is hydroxylated to 25-OH cholecalciferol in the liver. *(REF. 2 — p. 228)*

240. A. Parathyroid hormone will mobilize calcium from the bone. *(REF. 2 — pp. 229–230)*

241. E. Obesity itself has not been associated with increased incidence of vitamin D deficiency. *(REF. 2 — p. 229)*

242. B. Oral administration of vitamin D (1,500 to 5,000 IU) will produce healing demonstrable within two to four weeks except in unusual cases of vitamin D-refractory rickets. Months or years may be required for complete healing, and in extreme instances complete repair may be impossible. *(REF. 2 — p. 229)*

243. C. In vitamin D deficiency, the cartilaginous cells of the epiphyseal plate fail to complete their normal cycle and there is patchy capillary penetration. *(REF. 2 — p. 229)*

244. A. An increase in phosphate decreases the absorption of calcium. *(REF. 2 — pp. 230–231)*

245. E. Parathyroid hormone causes increased calcium absorption from the intestine, and this action is enhanced by 1,25-hydroxycholecalciferol. *(REF. 2 — pp. 229–230)*

246. A. Calcitonin is secreted by the thyroid. *(REF. 2 — p. 230)*

247. E. All of the choices given except conjunctivitis are fairly early signs of rickets that occur after several months of vitamin D deficiency. *(REF. 2 — pp. 231–232)*

248. B. These are all easily recognized signs of advanced rickets. *(REF. 2 — pp. 231–232)*

249. C. The distal ends of the ulna and radius show characteristic changes at an early stage. *(REF. 2 — p. 232)*

250. B. This amount is present in 32 oz of either whole milk or a 13 oz can of evaporated milk. *(REF. 2 — p. 234)*

251. E. While it may be helpful and advisable in some cases to correct disturbances in Ca/P ratios in the diet, this alone will not be useful in the treatment of rickets. *(REF. 2 — p. 234)*

252. D. Hypercalcemia and hypercalciuria are notable. Differential diagnosis includes chronic nephritis, hyperparathyroidism, and idiopathic hypercalemia. *(REF. 2 — p. 235)*

253. D. Prematures have poor absorption of vitamin E and patients with malabsorption are at risk. The minimum daily requirement of vitamin E is not known but 1 mg per 0.6 gm of unsaturated fat in the diet appears adequate. Premature infants should receive at least 5 mg daily. *(REF. 2 — pp. 235-236)*

254. B. Vitamin K is effective in reducing the fall in prothrombin associated with large-dose salicylates. *(REF. 2 — p. 236)*

255. E. Enamel defects may be seen in the permanent teeth, and they are fairly common if the rickets was untreated for a prolonged period. *(REF. 2 — p. 201)*

256. C. Extracellular fluid volume is approximately 20% of body weight. *(REF. 2 — p. 262)*

257. A. ICF is calculated as the difference between total body water and extracellular water and amounts to about 30 to 40% of body weight in a child over one year of age. *(REF. 2 — p. 263)*

258. C. Urine volume is influenced by diet and can be reduced only to that necessary to excrete solute load. *(REF. 2 — p. 264)*

259. D. An increase in ECF osmolality in relation to that of the ICF will stimulate ADH secretion. The sodium remains predominantly in the ECF, increasing the osmolality in relation to that of ICF. *(REF. 2 — p. 264)*

260. A. Forty-three percent of total body sodium is present in bone, the majority of which is either slowly exchangeable or completely nonexchangeable. *(REF. 2 — p. 266)*

261. D. Absorption of sodium occurs throughout the gastrointestinal tract, maximally in the jejunum. *(REF. 2 — p. 267)*

262. D. Most intracellular potassium is unbound and osmotically active. *(REF. 2 — p. 270)*

263. D. Serum electrolyte values indicate the *relative* losses of water and electrolytes. Patients with Addison's disease will enter negative sodium balance because of inappropriately elevated urine sodium. Cushing's disease results in positive sodium balance because of increased steroid production with mineral corticoid effects. *(REF. 2 — pp. 269, 291)*

264. D. Sick infants should be provided with glucose to combat hypoglycemia. Potassium should be given only after renal function has been established. *(REF. 2 — p. 293)*

265. C. The child's intake of calories is very often substandard because of psychosocial circumstances that are not clear at first glance. *(REF. 2 — pp. 311–312)*

VI: Immunologic Disorders

DIRECTIONS: Each of the questions or incomplete statements below is followed by five suggested answers or completions. Select the **one** that is **BEST** in each case.

266. Which one of the following components within the immune system is LEAST likely to be protective against bacterial infection?
    A. T cell
    B. Macrophage
    C. B cell
    D. Complement
    E. Plasma cell

267. Which of the following classes of immunoglobulins is known to both cross the placental barrier and combine with complement?
    A. IgG
    B. IgM
    C. IgA
    D. IgE
    E. IgD

268. Which of the following, when cell bound and combined with specific antigens, may produce physiologic effects that result in clinical allergic symptomatology?
    A. IgG
    B. IgM
    C. IgA
    D. IgE
    E. IgD

269. Increased susceptibility to what type of infection occurs in splenectomized patients?

   A. Viral
   B. Fungal
   C. Gram-positive bacterial and nonpolysaccharide-containing organism
   D. Gram-negative bacterial and polysaccharide-containing organism
   E. Gram-positive bacterial and polysaccharide-containing organism

270. Which of the following is NOT associated with IgM?

   A. Normally not found in cord blood of newborns
   B. Produced, in part, in the spleen
   C. Has the longest biologic half-life of all the major immunoglobulins
   D. Comprises 5% to 10% of the total immunoglobulins under normal circumstances
   E. When elevated, usually represents a response to either intrauterine or neonatal infection

271. By what age has cellular immunity become established?

   A. 20 weeks gestation
   B. 25 weeks gestation
   C. 30 weeks gestation
   D. 35 weeks gestation
   E. 40 weeks gestation

272. Which one of the following statements is FALSE regarding cell-mediated immunity?

   A. Majority of peripheral blood lymphocytes of normal children are T cells
   B. Cell-mediated immunity is important in protection against bacterial infection
   C. Once sensitized to a specific antigen, a T cell will react on second exposure by either going into blast formation or by releasing lymphokines
   D. Lymphocytes may release interferon to specific antigens
   E. T cells are necessary for normal antibody production by B lymphocytes

273. Which of the following is the primary circulating phagocyte?
  A. Neutrophil
  B. Lymphocyte
  C. Macrophage
  D. Monocyte
  E. Plasma cell

274. Which of the following statements concerning the phagocytic system is FALSE?
  A. Prior to phagocytosis, foreign antigens such as bacteria must interact with serum proteins
  B. Opsonins are composed primarily of immunoglobulins of IgM class
  C. Ingestion of a foreign particle is an active process requiring ATP, glycolysis, and glycogenolysis
  D. Chemotactic factors are released from bacteria following activation of the complement system
  E. Tissue phagocytes are primarily macrophages

275. Steroids inhibit phagocytosis by all of the following mechanisms EXCEPT
  A. by increasing intracellular levels of cyclic AMP
  B. by inhibiting glycolysis
  C. by increasing intracellular levels of cyclic GMP
  D. by impairing intracellular degranulation
  E. by decreasing intracellular levels of cyclic AMP

276. Which of the following may NOT activate the complement system?
  A. Properdin
  B. Antigen-antibody complexes
  C. Polysaccharide
  D. IgA
  E. Lysosomal enzymes

277. On laboratory screening, which of the following usually denotes immunodeficiency?
  A. IgG level less than 200 mg/dl
  B. IgM level of 10 mg/dl
  C. Positive Schick test in a completely immunized patient
  D. Total lymphocyte count at any age of 1,200/mm^3
  E. IgA level less than 10 mg/dl

92 / Immunologic Disorders

278. Depression of T-cell rosettes, as a quantitative in vitro measure of circulating T lymphocytes, is seen in all of the following EXCEPT
    A. acute and chronic viral infection
    B. malignancy
    C. infectious mononucleosis
    D. autoimmune disease
    E. cellular immunodeficiency disorders

279. Hypogammaglobulinemia resulting from a failure of B cells to synthesize and/or release immunoglobulins is called
    A. congenital
    B. acquired
    C. transient
    D. secondary
    E. chronic

280. Which of the following is NOT true regarding selective IgA deficiency?
    A. Patients usually have increased incidence of autoimmune disease
    B. Normal or increased levels of other immunoglobulins
    C. Usually have serum levels of 10 mg/dl
    D. Usually have absent salivary IgA
    E. Secretory IgA is absent in majority

281. Which of the following statements does NOT characterize neutropenia?
    A. Generally poor prognosis
    B. Number of circulating neutrophils less than 1,200/mm^3
    C. May be due to an isoimmune phonomenon following placental passage of antibodies directed against infant's neutrophils
    D. Infections fequent but usually not severe
    E. May have recurrent aphthous ulcers and/or stomatitis

282. Which one of the following is NOT characteristic of disorders following splenectomy?
  A. Increased susceptibility to infection with polysaccharide-containing organisms
  B. Splenectomy in patient with Wiskott-Aldrich syndrome is uniformly fatal
  C. Presence of adequate number of opsonins in form of antibody is important prognostic factor
  D. Age at splenectomy is not an important consideration
  E. Patients with sickle cell disease have increased susceptibility to pneumococcal infections

283. Lazy leukocyte syndrome is associated with all of the following EXCEPT
  A. defective phagocytic response to normal chemotactic stimuli
  B. normal number of neutrophils
  C. normal humoral and cellular immunity
  D. recurrent low-grade fever, gingivitis, stomatitis, and otitis media
  E. in vitro leukocyte phagocytosis and bacterial killing are normal

284. Which of the following statements concerning chronic granulomatous disease is FALSE?
  A. Basic defect in WBC is deficient respiratory oxidative metabolic activity
  B. Organisms commonly associated with this disease include streptococci and pneumococci
  C. Polymorphonuclear leukocytes normally phagocytize but are defective in bactericidal function
  D. It is inherited primarily as a sex-linked recessive trait
  E. It is evidence of abnormal function of eosinophils and mononuclear phagocytic cells

285. Which one of the following is NOT characteristic of Chédiak-Steinbrinck-Higashi syndrome?
  A. Hepatosplenomegaly
  B. CNS abnormalities
  C. Abnormal killing of streptococci, pneumococci, and staphylococci by WBC
  D. Sex-linked recessive inheritance
  E. Poor prognosis

DIRECTIONS: Each group of questions below consists of five lettered headings, followed by a list of numbered words, phrases or statements. For **each** numbered word, phrase or statement, select the **one** lettered heading that is most closely associated with it. Each lettered heading may be selected once, more than once, or not at all.

A. Chédiak-Steinbrinck-Higashi syndrome
B. Ataxia-telangiectasia
C. Wiskott-Aldrich syndrome
D. DiGeorge syndrome
E. Nezelof syndrome

286. Sex-linked recessive

287. Abnormality in granulocyte morphology

288. Associated with hypocalcemia in the neonatal period

289. Cellular immunodeficiency and normal immunoglobulin levels with specific antibody production absent

290. Autosomal recessive disorder with IgA deficiency

291. Associated with neonatal thrombocytopenia

A. IgA
B. IgM
C. IgG
D. IgD
E. IgE

292. Crosses the placenta

293. Binding sites for this globulin can be found on mast cells

294. Found primarily in secretions

295. Immunoglobulin with the lowest serum concentration

296. High concentrations are found in colostrum

297. Adult coverage serum concentration 150 mg/dl but absent in cord blood

A. T cell
B. B cell
C. Polymorphonuclear leukocyte
D. Kupffer cell
E. Plasma cell

298. Produces the majority of circulating immunoglobulins *E*

299. Absent in DiGeorge syndrome *A*

300. Main defective cell in chronic granulomatous disease *C*

301. Noncirculating macrophage *D*

302. Main element of cell-mediated immunity *A*

303. Makes up 20% to 30% of the circulating lymphocytes *B*

VI: Immunologic Disorders Answers and Comments

266. A. All of the other components actively participate in action against bacterial infection. *(REF. 1 — p. 299)*

267. A. IgM does not cross the placenta but does bind complement. IgA, IgD, and IgE neither actively cross the placenta nor bind complement. *(REF. 1 — p. 300)*

268. D. Histamine, SRS-A, and eosinophilic chemotactic factor may be released. *(REF. 1 — p. 301)*

269. D. The spleen probably has an important role in the production of IgM antibody, which forms against polysaccharides and against gram-negative bacterial antigens. *(REF. 1 — p. 301)*

270. C. IgG has the longest half-life of the major immunoglobulins (25 days). IgM has a half-life of only five days. *(REF. 1 — p. 300)*

271. A. Cellular immunity has become established by this age, since birth cells from thymus have already been distributed as competent T cells throughout the lymphoreticular system. *(REF. 1 — p. 301)*

272. B. Cell-mediated immunity is important in protection against viral, fungal, and protozoan infections. *(REF. 1 — p. 302)*

273. A. The macrophage and subsequently the monocyte reside in the tissue. Lymphocytes are not primarily circulating phagocytes. *(REF. 1 — p. 302)*

274. B. Opsonins are composed primarily of immunoglobulins of IgG class. *(REF. 1 — p. 302)*

275. C. Steroids increase levels of cyclic GMP which enhance intracellular degranulation and hence insure phagocytosis. *(REF. 1 — p. 303)*

276. D. IgA does not bind complement. *(REF. 1 — pp. 300, 303)*

277. C. Normal antibody will neutralize diphtheria toxin, and no reaction will be seen following skin testing with Schick reagent. *(REF. 1 — p. 305)*

278. C. Elevated levels of T-cell rosettes have been described in infectious mononucleosis. *(REF. 1 — p. 307)*

279. B. Congenital hypogammaglobulinemia usually lacks identifiable B cells in the peripheral blood. Transient hypogammaglobulinemia usually results in delay in production of immunoglobulin and the secondary form is most frequent in protein-losing states. *(REF. 1 — p. 309)*

280. C. Patients with selective IgA deficiency have less than 5 mg/dl of serum A and normal or increased levels of other immunoglobulins. *(REF. 1 — p. 311)*

281. A. Good prognosis may be possible because patients are usually able to mobilize monocytes in a compensatory manner. *(REF. 1 — p. 323)*

282. D. Age is a very critical consideration; in fact, splenectomized infants probably should receive antibiotics prophylactically. *(REF. 1 — p. 323)*

283. B. Neutropenia is characteristic of this disorder. *(REF. 1 — p. 323)*

284. B. Streptococci and pneumococci contain hydrogen peroxide which supplies the defective WBC with this necessary killing ingredient. Chronic granulomatous disease is often accompanied by bacterial infection caused by *Serratia marcescens* or *Staphylococcus epidermis*. *(REF. 1 — p. 324)*

285. D. The Chédiak-Steinbrinck-Higashi syndrome is transmitted by autosomal recessive gene. *(REF. 1 — p. 325)*

286. C. Wiskott-Aldrich syndrome is the only sex-linked disorder
287. A. listed and is associated with neonatal thrombocytopenia.
288. D. DiGeorge syndrome consists of thymic and parathyroid
289. E. aplasia and can present with neonatal hypocalcemia. The
290. B. ataxia-telangiectasia syndrome most commonly exhibits

291. C. IgA deficiency and is autosomal recessive. Chédiak-Steinbrinck-Higashi syndrome is also autosomal recessive but
has no associated IgA abnormality. It does however have an associated dysmorphology of the granulocytes (giant cytoplasmic granular inclusions). Nezelof syndrome is a primary immunodeficiency
disease characterized by varying degrees of cellular immunodeficiency and normal or nearly normal immunoglobulin levels. *(REF. 1
— pp. 314–325)*

292. C. IgM does not cross the placenta and is normally absent in
293. E. cord blood, while the adult level is 150 mg/dl. IgE binds to
294. A. mast cells and is the immunoglobulin with the lowest
295. E. serum concentration. IgA is found primarily in secretions
296. A. and the extravascular space. IgG does cross the placenta
297. B. and is the immunoglobulin with the highest serum concentration at birth. *(REF. 1 — p. 300)*

298. E. The T-cell lymphocyte is programmed from the thymus
299. A. and is absent in the DiGeorge syndrome (2° to thymic
300. C. aplasia). This is the main element of cell-mediated im-
301. D. munity. The majority of circulating immunoglobulins are
302. A. produced by the plasma cell, which is derived from the B
303. B. cell. Both Kupffer cells and polys are macrophages, but
the Kupffer cell is a tissue macrophage while the poly circulates. The main defect in chronic granulomatous disease is in the
bacterial lysing ability of the poly. *(REF. 1 — p. 299)*

VII: Allergy

DIRECTIONS: Each of the questions or incomplete statements below is followed by five suggested answers or completions. Select the one that is **BEST** in each case.

---

304. Which of the following classes of hypersensitivity reactions best fits the statement: Neither antigen nor antibody is coupled to a target-cell surface; rather, complexes of free antigen and antibody are circulating, and they either form microprecipitates in vessels or tissue fluid or they are free in antigen excess–toxic complex form?
    - **A.** Type I (anaphylactic-atopic) reaction
    - **B.** Type II (cytolytic or cytotoxic) reaction
    - **C.** Type III (Arthus) reaction
    - **D.** Type IV (cellular immune or delayed hypersensitivity) reaction
    - **E.** None of the above

305. Which of the following classes of hypersensitivity reactions best fits the statement: Serum antibodies are not involved and this reaction cannot be passively transferred with serum?
    - **A.** Type I
    - **B.** Type II
    - **C.** Type III
    - **D.** Type IV
    - **E.** None of the above

306. Which of the following combinations best describes the situation in Type I (anaphylactic-atopic) reactions regarding antibody formation?
A. IgG, IgM
B. IgG, IgE
C. IgM, IgE
D. IgG, IgM, IgA
E. IgG, IgM, IgA, IgD, or IgE

307. Which of the following combinations of antibodies may be produced by hyposensitization and be considered as blocking antibodies?
A. IgG, IgA
B. IgG, IgM
C. IgG, IgE
D. IgA, IgE
E. IgA, IgD

308. Which of the following drugs prevents metabolic degradation of cyclic AMP by inactivation of phosphodiesterases, which causes a rise in smooth muscle cyclic AMP and relaxation of bronchial smooth muscle?
A. Theophylline
B. Epinephrine
C. Propranolol
D. Norepinephrine
E. Terbutaline

309. Which of the following drug combinations of beta-adrenergic blockers enhances the release of histamine?
A. Theophylline, epinephrine
B. Epinephrine, isoproterenol
C. Propranolol, norepinephrine
D. Theophylline, isoproterenol
E. Propranolol, epinephrine

310. Which of the following drugs converts inactive adenylate cyclase into active adenylate cyclase, which in turn catalyzes the conversion of ATP to cyclic AMP causing bronchial smooth muscle relaxation?
  A. Theophylline
  B. Epinephrine
  C. Propranolol
  D. Norepinephrine
  E. Isoproterenol

311. Which of the following statements does NOT accurately describe childhood asthma?
  A. The intrinsic form is more common than the extrinsic
  B. It represents the classic form of Type I immediate hypersensitivity
  C. IgE antibodies are increased
  D. It is associated with the release of slow-reacting substance of anaphylaxis
  E. Between attacks the patient may appear symptomatically well

312. Which of the following progressions best describes status asthmaticus?
  A. Respiratory acidemia, respiratory alkalemia, metabolic acidemia
  B. Respiratory alkalemia, respiratory acidemia, metabolic acidemia
  C. Respiratory acidemia, metabolic acidemia, respiratory alkalemia
  D. Respiratory alkalemia, metabolic acidemia, respiratory acidemia
  E. Respiratory alkalemia, metabolic alkalemia, respiratory acidemia

313. Which of the following is considered the main mediator in angioedema?
  A. Histamine
  B. Bradykinin
  C. Prostaglandin E_1
  D. Serotonin
  E. SRS-A

314. Which of the following combinations is considered the primary mediator in anaphylaxis?
   A. Histamine, SRS-A
   B. SRS-A, prostaglandin E
   C. Serotonin, bradykinin
   D. Serotonin, histamine
   E. Histamine, bradykinin

315. Of the following types of hypersensitivity responses, which may be associated with drug allergy?
   A. Type I (anaphylactic-atopic)
   B. Type II (cytolytic or cytotoxic)
   C. Type III (Arthus reaction)
   D. Type IV (cellular immune or delayed hypersensitivity)
   E. All of the above

316. Which of the following statements does NOT characterize penicillin allergy?
   A. The metabolic pathway for major determinants is responsible for most anaphylactic reactions
   B. Rash and symptoms like those of serum sickness are caused by IgE antibodies to major pathway products
   C. With large amounts of penicillin, RBC membranes become coated with penicillin G and are recognized as being foreign and then are lysed
   D. Any of the four types of hypersensitivity response may occur
   E. Blocking antibody can be formed

VII: Allergy
Answers and Comments

304. C. In the Arthus reaction, antigen and IgG or IgM antibody at optimal proportions form microprecipitates in capillaries. *(REF. 1 — p. 330)*

305. D. Although delayed hypersensitivity cannot be passively transferred with serum, passive transfer of sensitized lymphocytes does cause cellular immune responses in the recipients upon contact with the antigen. *(REF. 1 — p. 330)*

306. E. Upon first exposure to an antigen, the individual responds by forming antibody that may be any one of the five classes. *(REF. 1 — p. 329)*

307. B. These antibodies have a neutralizing capacity that intercepts allergens on subsequent exposure and neutralizes the antigen in the circulation or tissues. These complexes are phagocytized and destroyed, thus preventing the antigen from reaching the IgE antibodies fixed to the surfaces of most cells and basophils. *(REF. 1 — p. 332)*

308. A. The beta-adrenergic agonist epinephrine inhibits the release of histamine and SRS-A from lung mast cells, whereas alpha-adrenergic stimulation by norepinephrine enhances these mediators. Further enhancement of histamine release occurs with administration of the beta-adrenergic blocker propranolol along with norepinephrine. *(REF. 1 — p. 334)*

309. C. Epinephrine and isoproterenol are beta-adrenergic agonists and inhibit release of histamine. Theophylline, especially when combined with epinephrine, inhibits histamine release. *(REF. 1 — p. 335)*

310. B. Epinephrine, a beta-adrenergic drug, acts at the earliest stage of the sympathetic system in converting adenylate cyclase to its active form. This active form in turn catalyzes the formation of cyclic AMP from ATP. *(REF. 1 — p. 334)*

311. A. Intrinsic asthma is more commonly seen in adults. *(REF. 1 — p. 346)*

312. B. Initially, respiratory alkalemia occurs as a result of hyperventilation, which is followed by increasing respiratory difficulty, CO_2 retention, and respiratory acidemia. Later, metabolic acidemia is superimposed as lactic acid and ketones accumulate from starvation and muscular effort. *(REF. 1 — p. 348)*

313. B. Histamine is the primary mediator in urticaria. Prostaglandin E_1 causes strong cutaneous vasodilation. SRS-A and serotonin increase vascular permeability in animals. *(REF. 1 — p. 358)*

314. E. The mechanism of anaphylaxis is a type I, IgE antibody-mediated reaction in which the allergen combines with IgE antibody on the surface of mast cells. This causes release of mediators, primarily histamine and bradykinin. *(REF. 1 — p. 360)*

315. E. Any of the four types of hypersensitivity responses may occur with drug allergy. *(REF. 1 — p. 364)*

316. A. The major penicilloyl determinant causes the formation of IgG antibodies in recently treated patients. These antibodies appear to act as blocking antibodies and prevent IgE-mediated anaphylactic reaction. Because large amounts of antigen are required for formation of IgG antibodies, blocking antibodies to minor determinants do not occur. *(REF. 1 — p. 364)*

VIII: Collagen Vascular Disorders

DIRECTIONS: Each of the questions or incomplete statements below is followed by five suggested answers or completions. Select the one that is BEST in each case.

---

317. The acute systemic form of juvenile rheumatoid arthritis (JRA) is characterized by all of the following EXCEPT
    A. it accounts for 50% of children with JRA
    B. it is associated with high fever and chills
    C. acute symptoms may precede joint symptoms by as much as six months
    D. a salmon-colored morbilliform rash
    E. hepatosplenomegaly is seen in approximately one-third of cases

318. The monoarticular form of JRA is characterized by all of the following EXCEPT
    A. it accounts for approximately 30% of cases of JRA
    B. iridocyclitis is a significant systemic manifestation and occurs in as many as 25% of patients
    C. small joints are commonly involved
    D. fatigue and low-grade fever are not prominent symptoms
    E. painless swelling of the joints is common

319. Polyarticular JRA is characterized by all of the following EXCEPT
  A. involvement of multiple joints, including fingers and toes
  B. systemic manifestations, including iridocyclitis, which are rare
  C. severe pain, erythema, and warmth, which are very common
  D. usually symmetrical joint involvement, with the large joints involved first
  E. limitation of joint motion, which occurs early

320. Which of the following statements regarding laboratory studies in JRA is true?
  A. ESR is frequently normal in all forms of JRA
  B. In a child with monoarticular arthritis, there is an increased likelihood of development of eye disease with a positive antinuclear antibody titer
  C. The majority of children with acute systemic JRA have normal WBC during active disease
  D. Rheumatoid factor is commonly positive
  E. Positive rheumatoid factor and antinuclear antibody titer in the same patient are pathognomonic of JRA

321. Which of the following does NOT characterize systemic lupus erythematosus?
  A. Tests for autoantibodies are frequently positive
  B. Family members of patients with SLE have increased incidence of hypergammaglobulinemia, rheumatoid factor, and ANA
  C. Skin manifestations of SLE without systemic disease are common in children
  D. Severe arthritis is present only infrequently, and deforming arthritis is rare
  E. Renal involvement is common at some time during the course of the disease

322. Which of the following statements regarding laboratory tests does NOT characterize SLE?
   A. Antinuclear antibody (ANA) is the single most important test
   B. ANA is a specific test for SLE
   C. LE preparation is less frequently positive in children than adults
   D. A positive LE prep is more specific for the diagnosis of SLE than is a positive ANA test
   E. Creatinine clearance is a useful indicator of the severity of renal involvement

323. All of the following are major criteria in the diagnosis of dermatomyositis in childhood EXCEPT
   A. progressive symmetric weakness of peripheral muscle groups
   B. evidence of necrosis of type I and type II muscle fibers
   C. elevation of skeletal muscle enzymes in serum
   D. characteristic heliotrope rash with periorbital edema
   E. scaly erythematous rash over dorsum of the hands

324. Which of the following is NOT associated with Henoch-Schönlein purpura?
   A. Nonthrombocytopenic purpura
   B. Gastrointestinal hemorrhage
   C. Arthralgia or mild arthritis
   D. Abdominal pain
   E. Poor prognosis

325. Which of the following tests is specific for acute rheumatic fever?
   A. Elevated ESR
   B. Elevated ASO titer
   C. Positive throat culture for Group A streptococci
   D. Prolonged P-R interval on EKG
   E. None of the above

326. Which of the following tests would provide the most reliable information in the diagnosis of acute rheumatic fever?
    A. ESR
    B. ECG P-R interval
    C. C-reactive protein
    D. ASO
    E. CBC

DIRECTIONS: For each of the questions or incomplete statements below, **ONE** or **MORE** of the answers or completions given is correct. Select

   A if only *1, 2 and 3* are correct,
   B if only *1 and 3* are correct,
   C if only *2 and 4* are correct,
   D if only *4* is correct,
   E if all are correct.

---

327. In the polyarticular form of juvenile rheumatoid arthritis
    1. mostly boys are affected
    2. any joint can be affected
    3. positive rheumatoid factor is less likely than other forms
    4. iridocyclitis is rare

328. The patient with ankylosing spondylitis
    1. has loss of lumbodorsal spine mobility and lower back pain during the course of the disease
    2. may have HLA W27
    3. usually has a good prognosis for functional outcome
    4. usually has a positive rheumatoid factor

329. In systemic lupus erythematosus
    1. anti-DNA antibodies are common
    2. steroids have no place in treatment
    3. immune complexes deposit in the nephron
    4. serum C3 determinations are of little value

330. Henoch-Schönlein syndrome (anaphylactoid purpura) may be characterized by
  1. arthritis, with or without effusion
  2. gastrointestinal bleeding
  3. variable skin rash
  4. renal involvement that may progress to chronic renal disease

331. The major clinical features of dermatomyositis include
  1. arthritis
  2. a scaly erythematous rash over the dorsum of the hands
  3. gallstones
  4. muscle weakness

332. Of the following, the diseases whose underlying defect is classified as a vasculitis include
  1. Wegener's granulomatosis
  2. Stevens-Johnson syndrome
  3. anaphylactoid purpura
  4. Sjögren's syndrome

333. Major manifestations of rheumatic fever according to the Jones criteria include
  1. carditis
  2. chorea
  3. polyarthritis
  4. increased ASO or other streptococcal antibodies

334. Signs of rheumatic carditis include
  1. prolongation of P-R interval
  2. bradycardia
  3. friction rub
  4. loud first heart sound

335. Clinical manifestations of systemic lupus erythematosus include
  1. hepatitis
  2. nephritis
  3. iritis
  4. psychosis

Directions Summarized				
A	B	C	D	E
1,2,3	1,3	2,4	4	All are
only	only	only	only	correct

336. Patients with the Goodpasture syndrome
    1. are usually young adult males
    2. usually die within a short period of time
    3. have intra-alveolar hemorrhages with hemosiderin-laden macrophages
    4. have a characteristic skin rash

VIII: Collagen Vascular Disorders
Answers and Comments

317. A. The acute systemic form of juvenile rheumatoid arthritis accounts for approximately 20% of the cases. *(REF. 1 — p. 374)*

318. C. Knees, ankles, and elbows are the joints most commonly involved. Small joints of hands are conspicuously spared. *(REF. 1 — p. 374)*

319. C. Severely painful, red, and hot joints are unusual in polyarticular JRA. *(REF. 1 — p. 374)*

320. B. ESR and WBCs are frequently normal in patients with monoarticular, pauciarticular, and polyarticular arthritis but are elevated in the majority of children with acute systemic JRA. Rheumatoid factor is rarely positive in children with JRA. *(REF. 1 — p. 374)*

321. C. Discord lupus is rare in children. *(REF. 1 — p. 377)*

322. B. A positive test for ANA may be present in chronic active hepatitis, Sjögren's syndrome, and rarely JRA. *(REF. 1 — p. 378)*

323. A. Muscle weakness is found in the limb-girdle groups and anterior neck flexors. *(REF. 1 — p. 380)*

324. E. Even with renal involvement, most children recover. *(REF. 1 — p. 382)*

325. E. None of these tests are specific for ARF. *(REF. 1 — p. 386)*

326. D. ESR elevation is nonspecific; P-R interval is present in over 20% of patients but lacks specificity; C-reactive protein is also nonspecific. One must have supportive evidence of recent streptococcal infection. *(REF. 1 — p. 386)*

327. C. Polyarticular arthritis is seen mainly in girls and is only rarely associated with iridocyclitis. Any joint can be affected, and of all the forms of JRA the rheumatoid factor is more frequently positive in the polyarticular form. *(REF. 2 — p. 653)*

328. A. Ankylosing spondylitis characteristically involves the lumbodorsal spine and sacroiliac joint. Patients frequently are found to be HLA W27 positive and this has been used as a marker of the disease. The long-term prognosis is usually good if posture is maintained. The rheumatoid factor is rarely positive. *(REF. 2 — pp. 663–664)*

329. B. Systemic lupus erythematosus is an autoimmune disease in which anti-DNA antibodies are formed, and renal immune complex deposition occurs. Only rarely may patients with SLE be managed without steroids. The level of serum C3 is a valuable guide to the activity of the disease. *(REF. 1 — p. 378)*

330. E. Anaphylactoid purpura is a syndrome that may include: arthritis with or without effusion, GI bleeding, a variable skin rash, and nephritis that can progress to chronic renal disease in some patients. *(REF. 2 — p. 671)*

331. C. Dermatomyositis can present with generalized muscle weakness. A scaly erythematous rash on the dorsum of the hands and knuckles is considered by some to be pathognomonic. Overt arthritis is rare and gallstones, if present, represent unrelated disease. *(REF. 1 — p. 381)*

332. E. Vasculitis is the hallmark of many rheumatic disease. Those in particular include Wegener's granulomatosis, H-S purpura, and the Stevens-Johnson syndrome. Sjögren's syndrome may have many of the features of polyarteritis. *(REF. 2 — p. 670)*

333. A. Based on the Jones criteria the major manifestations of rheumatic fever include carditis, polyarthritis, chorea, erythema marginatum, and subcutaneous nodules. Streptococcal antibodies are considered supportive evidence of a recent strep infection. Supportive evidence of a recent strep infection must accompany the manifestations of disease before a diagnosis can be made. *(REF. 1 — p. 385)*

334. B. The manifestations of rheumatic carditis include the evidence of pericarditis (friction rub), cardiomegaly, and prolongation of the P-R interval (among others). Bradycardia and a loud S1 are not signs of carditis. *(REF. 1 — p. 388)*

335. E. The clinical manifestations of SLE are the result of the widespread vasculitis that accompanies this disorder. The liver (hepatitis), eye (iritis), brain (psychosis), and kidney (nephritis) are all involved. *(REF. 2 — p. 667)*

336. A. Patients with the Goodpasture syndrome usually die after a rapid downhill course. They are usually young adult males and at autopsy are found to have intra-alveolar hemorrhages and hemosiderin-laden macrophages. There is no characteristic skin rash. *(REF. 2 — p. 679)*

IX: Bacterial and Viral Infections

DIRECTIONS: Each of the questions or incomplete statements below is followed by five suggested answers or completions. Select the **one** that is **BEST** in each case.

---

337. Endotoxin is characterized by all of the following EXCEPT
    A. it is a lipopolysaccharide component of the outer membrane of the organism
    B. it may promote a consumption coagulopathy by activating the clotting sequence
    C. it fixes complement directly via the alternate pathway
    D. it produces hypothermia
    E. it is one of the main surface antigens of gram-negative organisms

338. All of the following statements regarding bacterial cell membranes are true EXCEPT
    A. they are composed mainly of protein
    B. membranes of different bacteria are antigenically distinct
    C. composition differs mainly from mammalian cells by the absence of sterols and by the types of phosphatides in the lipids
    D. penicillin acts primarily against bacterial membrane
    E. they are composed of about 40% lipid and 60% protein

339. Which of the following drugs acts against bacterial cell wall?
    A. Penicillin
    B. Polymyxin B
    C. Rifampin
    D. Chloramphenicol
    E. Gentamicin

340. Which of the following antibiotics interferes with protein synthesis of bacteria?
    A. Penicillin
    B. Aminoglycoside
    C. Sulfonamide
    D. Bacitracin
    E. Polymyxin B

341. Which of the following drugs affects intermediary metabolism of bacteria?
    A. Sulfonamide
    B. Penicillin
    C. Erythromycin
    D. Chloramphenicol
    E. Cephalosporin

342. The antibacterial activity of which of the following drugs is most affected by pH?
    A. Vancomycin
    B. Sulfonamide
    C. Bacitracin
    D. Aminoglycoside
    E. Oxacillin

343. Which of the following is NOT associated with carbenicillin?
    A. It is destroyed by penicillinase
    B. Activity is increased by alkaline pH
    C. It obtains high concentration in urinary tract
    D. It has synergistic antibacterial activity when combined with gentamicin against most strains of *Pseudomonas*
    E. It is a disodium molecule

344. Which of the following statements is FALSE regarding lincomycin?
    A. It is active against anaerobic bacteria
    B. It actively penetrates into the cerebrospinal fluid
    C. Diarrhea and GI upset are common
    D. It is similar to erythromycin in absorption and spectrum of action
    E. It is bacteriostatic

345. Chloramphenicol is associated with all of the following EXCEPT
    A. it is well absorbed from GI tract and diffuses well into CSF
    B. idiosyncratic reaction causing aplastic anemia is dose related
    C. it is conjugated in the liver with glucuronide
    D. it is effective against many *Rickettsia* but not against *Pseudomonas*
    E. it is bacteriostatic

346. The organism most commonly associated with neonatal bacterial disease is
    A. *Staphylococcus aureus*
    B. Group B beta-hemolytic streptococci
    C. *Listeria monocytogenes*
    D. *Escherichia coli*
    E. *Pseudomonas*

347. The most common bacterial organism associated with meningitis in infants and children is
    A. *Diplococcus pneumoniae*
    B. *Neisseria meningitidis*
    C. Group A beta-hemolytic streptococcus
    D. *Haemophilus influenzae*
    E. Group B beta-hemolytic streptococcus

348. Which of the following statements does NOT characterize bacterial meningitis in young infants?
    A. Only specific feature may be bulging of the anterior fontanelle
    B. Nuchal rigidity is commonly present
    C. *H. influenzae* is the most common organism
    D. Papilledema is rarely seen
    E. Poor feeding is common

349. Viral meningitis is characterized by all of the following EX-CEPT
   A. CSF cell count may show transient predominance in polymorphonuclear WBCs early in the course
   B. CSF sugar is elevated
   C. CSF protein may be moderately elevated
   D. CSF findings are similar to lead encephalitis
   E. predominant cytology is mononuclear

350. Subdural effusions complicating meningitis are associated with all of the following EXCEPT
   A. extremely rare in meningococcal meningitis
   B. persistent vomiting recurring after initial clinical improvement
   C. most commonly accompany infection caused by *H. influenzae* and *D. pneumoniae*
   D. patients frequently show signs of cerebral damage
   E. recovery of 2 ml or more of xanthochromic fluid with a protein content exceeding by 40 mg that of the spinal fluid

351. All of the following characterize infection with *Clostridium botulinum* EXCEPT
   A. toxic effects arise at the myoneural junction by preventing the release of acetylcholine
   B. there is no known pharmacologic antagonist
   C. symptoms usually develop rapidly after ingestion
   D. patients are usually afebrile and mentally alert
   E. it is usually a result of foods improperly prepared at home

352. Infection with *Brucella* is characterized by all of the following EXCEPT
   A. it is usually associated with ingestion of infected milk products or direct contact with dogs
   B. organisms in the human body are usually disseminated to reticuloendothelial system
   C. prognosis is usually poor
   D. it cross reacts serologically with *Francisella tularensis*
   E. the incubation period is usually five to 30 days

353. Concerning the infection due to *Corynebacterium diphtheriae*, which of the following statements is FALSE?
   A. Myocarditis is a common lesion and the changes are degenerative rather than inflammatory
   B. Bacteria usually remain on surface lesions of respiratory systems and rarely cause bacteremia
   C. Complications due to the toxins may occur as late as six weeks after the initial infection
   D. Primary nasal involvement is usually seen in older children and adults
   E. Incubation period is usually between two to five days

354. Infection with which of the following is LEAST likely to be confused with the pseudomembrane of diphtheria?
   A. Epstein-Barr virus
   B. Group A beta-hemolytic streptococcus
   C. Vincent's organisms
   D. Adenovirus
   E. Toxoplasmosis

355. The most common manifestation of disseminated gonorrhea in adolescents and adults is
   A. myocarditis
   B. meningitis
   C. hemorrhagic skin lesions
   D. pyelonephritis
   E. arthritis

356. Which of the following statements is FALSE regarding gonococcal infections?
   A. Prior infections usually confer protective immunity
   B. Associated with production of local and systemic antibody as well as cell-mediated response
   C. Predilection for infecting mucosal surfaces lined by columnar as opposed to stratified epithelium
   D. pH of vaginal mucus and thickness of mucosa are important modifiers in susceptibility to infection
   E. Symptoms usually appear within one week of infection

357. Infection with *H. influenzae* is characterized by all of the following EXCEPT
    A. it is the most common bacterial meningitis in young children
    B. synergy with certain respiratory viruses may be important in colonization production of local respiratory disease
    C. 95% of invasive strains are type B
    D. the nonencapsulated organism is associated with disease more often than the encapsulated form
    E. facial cellulitis is more common than pyarthrosis

358. Bacteremia in children is most often associated with which of the following organisms?
    A. *H. influenzae*
    B. Pneumococcus
    C. Hemolytic streptococcus
    D. *S. aureus*
    E. *E. coli*

359. The most common location of *H. influenzae* cellulitis is the
    A. limbs
    B. trunk
    C. face
    D. periorbital area
    E. external auditory canal

360. Acute epiglottitis due to *H. influenzae* type B is characterized by all of the following EXCEPT
    A. sore throat
    B. dysphagia with pooling of secretions
    C. stridor
    D. position of ease is supine with chin extended
    E. fever

361. *H. influenzae* pyarthrosis is associated with all of the following EXCEPT
    A. it precedes upper respiratory infection
    B. multiple joint involvement
    C. no abnormalities of long bones
    D. a usually large weight bearing joint
    E. usually acutely ill and toxic

362. All of the following are associated with the first phase of septicemia secondary to infection with leptospirosis EXCEPT
  A. fever and headache
  B. myalgia
  C. meningitis
  D. gastrointestinal disturbances
  E. proteinuria

363. Which of the following is considered the most common presentation of meningococcal infection?
  A. Acute meningitis
  B. Maculopapular rash
  C. Petechial rash
  D. Gastroenteritis
  E. Splenomegaly

364. A differential diagnosis of meningococcal disease would include all of the following EXCEPT
  A. Coxsackie type A9 viral infection
  B. rickettsial disease
  C. ECHO viral infection
  D. atypical measles
  E. adenoviral infection

365. Which of the following is considered to be effective prophylaxis against meningococcal infections among close contacts?
  A. Penicillin
  B. Rifampin
  C. Sulfonamide
  D. Tetracycline
  E. Erythromycin

366. In infection with *Mycoplasma pneumoniae*, which of the following is generally FALSE?
  A. Peripheral leukocyte count is normal
  B. Rise in complement-fixing antibodies in two to three weeks
  C. Pulmonary lesions resemble miliary granuloma
  D. Child usually appears less ill than fever indicates
  E. ESR rises

367. Differential diagnosis of *M. pneumoniae,* other than bacterial organisms, would include all of the following EXCEPT
   A. respiratory syncytial virus (RSV)
   B. adenovirus
   C. influenza virus
   D. parainfluenza virus
   E. psittacosis virus

368. Which of the following is NOT considered characteristic of pertussis?
   A. May be seen early in life owing to a lack of maternal antibodies
   B. The catarrhal stage precedes the paroxysmal stage
   C. The paroxysmal cough may last for one to four weeks
   D. The peripheral WBC is usually significantly elevated with a shift to polymorphonuclear leukocytes
   E. Incubation period is between five and ten days

369. All of the following may be considered in the differential diagnosis of disease due to *Bordetella pertussis* EXCEPT
   A. *H. influenzae* type bronchitis
   B. interstitial pneumonitis due to respiratory syncytial virus
   C. infection with *B. parapertussis*
   D. infection with ECHO virus
   E. foreign body in bronchial airway

370. Disease due to *B. parapertussis* may be similar to that due to *B. pertussis* in all of the following EXCEPT
   A. cultural growth
   B. shared antigens but no cross-immunity
   C. clinical syndrome
   D. respiratory disease
   E. respiratory pathology

371. Regarding pathogenesis of tuberculosis, which of the following is FALSE?
    A. Tuberculin hypersensitivity develops in the host four to eight weeks after infection, and the skin test becomes positive
    B. The greatest risk for progression of primary complex with occurrence of meningitis and miliary disease is during the first 12 months after the primary infection
    C. Skeletal lesions appear within two to four years of the primary infection
    D. Renal lesions appear early within two to three years of the primary infection
    E. The nodal component of the primary complex shows less tendency to heal completely than the parenchymal focus

372. Primary tuberculosis is characterized by all of the following EXCEPT
    A. an incubation period of two to eight weeks
    B. the majority of cases are innocuous with healing and calcification of Ghon complex occurring as early as six months
    C. the most common symptoms of progressive disease are cough, fever, and night sweats
    D. involvement of bronchial wall by enlarging lymph nodes is a rare complication of primary complex
    E. the skin test is nonreactive for eight weeks after the initial infection

373. Which of the following does NOT characterize chronic pulmonary tuberculosis?
    A. The risk of developing this problem is greatest during adolescence
    B. Miliary tuberculosis is a complication of chronic tuberculosis
    C. Represents endogenous reinfection by previously established tuberculosis bacilli
    D. Chronic tuberculosis usually remains a pulmonary disease
    E. The clinical picture is that of respiratory infection

374. Tuberculous meningitis is characterized by all of the following EXCEPT
- **A.** it is the most serious complication of tuberculosis
- **B.** it results from metastatic disease during early occult hematogenous dissemination of primary infection
- **C.** it is always a meningoencephalitis
- **D.** CSF shows marked elevation of WBC
- **E.** the CSF glucose is normal early, but tends to decrease as the disease progresses

375. Which of the following is usually NOT associated with skeletal tuberculosis?
- **A.** Results from hematogenous dissemination early in course of primary infection
- **B.** Most common sites are hands and feet
- **C.** Dactylitis occurs almost solely in infants
- **D.** Bone and joint manifestations develop frequently within first year
- **E.** Spondylitis is unusual in small infants

376. Which of the following organisms is most often associated with lymphadenitis in children?
- **A.** *Mycobacterium kansasii*
- **B.** *Mycobacterium scrofulaceum*
- **C.** *Mycobacterium intracelluare*
- **D.** *Mycobacterium avium*
- **E.** *Mycobacterium bovis*

377. Which of the following organisms is LEAST often associated with superficial disease?
- **A.** *Mycobacterium marinum*
- **B.** *Mycobacterium ulcerans*
- **C.** *Mycobacterium intracellulare*
- **D.** *Mycobacterium fortuitum*
- **E.** *Mycobacterium scrofulaceum*

378. Which of the following statements regarding mycobacterial infection, other than *Mycobacterium tuberculosis,* is FALSE?
    A. Infection is not communicable in man
    B. Generally resistant to antitubercular treatment
    C. Usually associated with a weakly positive PPD or 5TU
    D. Pulmonary involvement is the most common manifestation of this disease in childhood
    E. Usually no history of tuberculosis in family

379. The treatment of choice for lymph node disease due to non-tubercular mycobacterial organism is
    A. complete excision
    B. isoniazid (INH)
    C. INH, para-aminosalicylic acid (PAS)
    D. rifampin
    E. ethambutol

380. Which of the following clinical forms of tularemia is most common?
    A. Ulceroglandular
    B. Pneumonic
    C. Oculoglandular
    D. Pharyngotonsillar
    E. Oropharyngeal

381. Which of the following is NOT considered characteristic of tularemia?
    A. Oropharyngeal disease is associated with a gray-white necrotic membrane
    B. The pneumonic form results from bacteremic spread to lungs
    C. Transmission from man to man
    D. Most common vector is tick
    E. Fever, myalgia, and headache may last as long as a month

382. The diagnosis of tularemia is characterized by all of the following EXCEPT
    A. skin test is sensitive and specific
    B. skin test induces agglutinins
    C. serum agglutination reaction is reliable but may show cross-reaction in patients with brucellosis
    D. WBC is often normal
    E. organism can be cultured from blood, sputum, exudates, and gastric washings

383. Which of the following does NOT characterize salmonellosis (nontyphoid fever)?
    A. The most common form is the gastroenteritic type
    B. In the *Salmonella paratyphi* form, rose spots, splenomegaly, and leukopenia may occur
    C. *Salmonella typhimurium* is the most common organism found in salmonella gastroenteritis
    D. Among the localized infections due to metastatic infection, meningitis is the most common
    E. Patients with sickle cell disease are particularly susceptible to osteomyelitis

384. Typhoid fever in infants and young children differs from that in older children and adults in all of the following EXCEPT
    A. peripheral WBC
    B. rose spots
    C. severity of disease
    D. association with *S. typhi*
    E. complications

385. Which of the following laboratory tests is NOT feasible in the diagnosis of shigellosis?
    A. Stool culture
    B. Blood culture
    C. Group and type-specific shigella antisera
    D. Search for blood and pus in stool specimens
    E. Demonstration of antibody responses

386. Which of the following is NOT characteristic of entero-pathogenic *E. coli* enteritis?
   A. Leukocytosis
   B. Watery stools
   C. Stools that contain neither blood nor pus
   D. Principle complications are secondary infections chiefly of the respiratory or urinary tract, the meninges, or the skin
   E. Intestinal mucosa usually shows no ulceration

387. Staphylococcal food poisoning is usually manifested by all of the following EXCEPT
   A. colicky abdominal pain
   B. little if any fever
   C. severe, watery mucoid diarrhea
   D. onset of symptoms a few hours after eating infected food
   E. it is rarely fatal

388. Group A beta-hemolytic streptococci differ from other groups in all of the following EXCEPT
   A. sensitivity to bacitracin
   B. specific carbohydrate antigen in cell wall
   C. involvement in initiating rheumatic fever and acute glomerulonephritis
   D. nonassociation with newborn infection
   E. association with a clear zone of hemolysis surrounding colonies grown on mammalian blood agar

389. Scarlet fever is associated with all of the following findings EXCEPT
   A. infection due to erythrogenic toxin-producing Group A beta-hemolytic streptococci
   B. punctate erythematous lesions on palate
   C. early onset (24 to 48 hours) of erythematous-punctiform rash
   D. heavy involvement of rash over face
   E. Pastia's lines

390. Group B beta-hemolytic streptococcal disease in the immediate newborn period differs from the delayed-onset disease in all of the following EXCEPT
   A. meningitis is the most common manifestation
   B. maternal factors are more common, i.e., premature labor, maternal perinatal fever
   C. mortality is higher in immediate period
   D. onset is more sudden
   E. clinical course is more rapid

391. Pathologic features that distinguish the syphilis of infancy and early childhood from that of later life include all of the following EXCEPT
   A. interstitial fibrosis of liver and spleen
   B. pneumonia consisting of increased connective tissue infiltrating the lung
   C. increased incidence of cardiovascular disease
   D. tissue alteration leading to allergic-type lesion such as interstitial keratitis
   E. scarring of lips and nose tissues

392. Which of the following is FALSE in regard to immunology and serodiagnosis of childhood syphilis?
   A. Maternal IgG may be transplacentally transmitted to the fetus
   B. Antibodies are of the IgM and IgG types
   C. Nonspecific antibody to syphilis may also be found in infectious mononucleosis, vaccinia, varicella, and SLE
   D. Transplacentally transferred antibody will produce a positive serologic test for syphilis (STS) but not a positive *Treponema pallidum* immobilization test (TPI)
   E. Transplacentally transferred antibody to the fetus may be equal to but not greater than the mothers

393. Regarding the epidemiology and etiology of cat-scratch disease (CSD), which of the following is FALSE?
   A. Occurs with the majority of cases in patients less than 20 years of age
   B. About 90% of those afflicted had contact with a cat
   C. Human to human transmissibility
   D. Cats do not react to skin tests with cat-scratch antigen
   E. Inoculation site is found in over half the patients

394. CSD is manifested by all of the following EXCEPT
   A. lymphadenopathy, the most common manifestation, which occurs most frequently in the head, neck, and axilla
   B. it should always be suspected in a patient with an ocular lesion and preauricular lymphadenitis
   C. thrombocytopenic purpura is a common sign
   D. an inoculation site (scratch or primary lesion) can be expected in at least 50% of affected patients
   E. suppuration of lymph nodes is uncommon

395. Which of the following statements regarding the etiology and epidemiology of chickenpox is FALSE?
   A. Caused by varicella zoster virus, which is a member of the poxvirus group
   B. Varicella is transmissible to man by inoculation of vesicular fluid from patients with either herpes zoster or varicella
   C. Subclinical infection rarely occurs
   D. Crusts of lesion do not contain viable viruses
   E. May occur in newborn period

396. Varicella is characterized by all of the following EXCEPT
   A. one attack usually confers lifelong immunity
   B. maternal varicella antibody is transplacentally passed when pregnant women get varicella
   C. incubation period ranges from 11 to 20 days
   D. if it occurs during first ten days of life it may result in disseminated infection
   E. varicella is generally much more severe in children than in adults

397. Which of the following is NOT characteristic of varicella?
   A. Lesions appear in crops over a period of three to five days
   B. Distribution of lesions is predominantly on the extremities as compared to the trunk
   C. The peripheral blood picture is essentially unchanged
   D. Primary varicella pneumonia is uncommon
   E. Prodromal period is mild, and symptoms may be absent

398. Smallpox can be differentiated from varicella by all of the following EXCEPT
    A. constitutional symptoms that precede the eruption of smallpox are severe, whereas with varicella they are worse at the height of the lesions
    B. smallpox lesions are all of uniform age and size in any one general area
    C. eruption of smallpox is usually centripetal
    D. modified smallpox may be clinically indistinguishable from varicella
    E. there are no intranuclear inclusions in cells prepared from the base of vesicles of smallpox as is the case with varicella

399. Congenital cytomegalovirus (CMV) is characterized by all of the following EXCEPT
    A. approximately 95% of infected infants are asymptomatic
    B. often the only physical finding is a general failure to thrive or increased irritability
    C. major complications of the infection are sequelae involving the CNS
    D. paraventricular cerebral calcification is more common than hepatosplenomegaly
    E. petechial rash on first day after birth is suggestive of disease

400. Which of the following is more characteristic of congenital rubella than of CMV?
    A. Purpuric rash
    B. Central cataracts
    C. Jaundice
    D. Microcephaly
    E. Deafness

401. Which of the following statements regarding acquired cytomegaloviral mononucleosis is FALSE?
    A. Atypical lymphocytosis is common
    B. May be associated with a maculopapular rash following ampicillin administration
    C. Usually heterophil antibody–positive
    D. The cytomegalovirus IgM (FA) test is positive in CMV and infectious mononucleosis presumably because EBV and CMV share common antigens
    E. Hepatomegaly and mildly abnormal liver function tests are found

402. Exanthema subitum (roseola infantum) is best distinguished from rubella by which of the following?
A. Height and duration of fever preceding the rash
B. Character of the rash
C. Location of lymphadenopathy
D. Peripheral WBC
E. Response to treatment

403. The most common viral agent associated with gastroenteritis in infants and young children is
A. ECHO virus
B. Rotavirus
C. Coxsackie virus
D. Norwalk virus
E. Coronavirus

404. Which of the following does NOT accurately characterize the clinical picture of viral hepatitis in children?
A. Onset is often abrupt
B. Anorexia and nausea and vomiting are common pre-icteric symptoms
C. Generalized jaundice most often precedes the color change in urine owing to excess bilirubin
D. Massive necrosis of hepatic parenchymal cells is rare
E. Constipation and diarrhea occur occasionally and with equal frequency

405. The most helpful laboratory test in the preicteric stage of viral hepatitis is
A. serum bilirubin
B. SGOT
C. prothrombin time
D. Bromsulphalein (BSP)
E. serum proteins

406. The most meaningful test in terms of severity and prognosis of viral hepatitis is
A. serum bilirubin
B. SGOT
C. serum proteins
D. BSP
E. prothrombin time

407. Which of the following is most significant in promoting recovery from viral hepatitis?
    A. Vitamin K
    B. Total caloric intake
    C. High-protein low-fat diet
    D. Supplemental B vitamins
    E. Bedrest

408. Which of the following statements differentiating type A hepatitis from type B hepatitis is FALSE?
    A. Onset is more abrupt with type A
    B. Fever is more frequent with type A
    C. Unapparent infections more common with type B
    D. Higher proportion of urticarial rashes and joint manifestations with type A
    E. Type B has been associated with and is presumably a cause of polyarteritis and glomerulonephritis

409. Which of the following statements is FALSE regarding hepatitis B surface antigen (HB_SAg) testing?
    A. Becomes positive one to two months prior to onset of symptoms
    B. A positive test for HB_SAg that becomes negative in convalescence is diagnostic of type B hepatitis
    C. Positive at onset of jaundice in majority of cases
    D. Positivity is not an index of carrier state
    E. Used as basis for screening blood donors for the carrier state

410. Hepatitis B virus can be transmitted from man to man by all of the following EXCEPT
    A. in urine
    B. in saliva
    C. transplacentally
    D. venereally
    E. in feces

411. Which of the following statements concerning the virology and epidemiology of herpes simplex virus (HSV) is FALSE?
   A. HSV type 2 primarily infects genital sites
   B. Recrudescences of infections occur in individuals with circulating HSV antibodies
   C. Infectious virus can be demonstrated in sensory ganglia
   D. Incubation period for neonates with herpetic infection is an average of one week
   E. Genital HSV-2 infection in pregnant women has been found to be the major source of virus for the newborn

412. The pathogenesis and immunity to HSV infections are characterized in part by all of the following EXCEPT
   A. primary infection is associated with more severe symptoms than in the case where acquired antibodies are present
   B. in recurrent HSV infections, neutralizing antibodies are present in all patients and these rise after each recurrence
   C. IgG, IgA, and IgM antibodies are present in the serum of patients with recurrent HSV infections
   D. depression of certain lymphokines may be correlated with increased predilection to HSV recurrence
   E. individuals with recurrence demonstrate positive responses to a variety of in vitro cell-mediated assays

413. Regarding the clinical manifestations of HSV infections, which of the following is FALSE?
   A. The oral cavity is the most common site of infection in children
   B. The lips are the most common site for HSV-1 recurrences but are infrequently the site for primary infection
   C. Eczema herpeticum is most often caused by a primary HSV infection
   D. The most common site of genital infection in females with HSV-2 is the labia
   E. Asymptomatic HSV infections in the newborn are infrequent

414. HSV infection of the CNS is characterized by all of the following EXCEPT
   A. most isolates from the brain of individuals beyond the newborn age are HSV-1
   B. HSV meningitis is primarily caused by HSV-1
   C. HSV meningitis is difficult to differentiate from other causes of aseptic meningitis
   D. brain biopsy is the only certain way to diagnose HSV encephalitis
   E. HSV-2 is more readily recoverable from the CSF than is HSV-1

415. The epidemiology of Epstein-Barr virus (EBV) infection is characterized by all of the following EXCEPT
   A. it is most often acquired during childhood
   B. infection usually occurs without clinically recognizable symptoms
   C. mononucleosis usually occurs during infection in adolescence and early adulthood
   D. there is a higher rate of infection among the upper socio-economic groups
   E. the role of reactivated virus in the genesis of the disease or in transmission has not yet been clarified

416. Infectious mononucleosis is clinically manifested by all of the following EXCEPT
   A. the classic picture is rarely seen in toddlers and young children infected with EBV
   B. heterophil agglutination is sometimes not detected in young children
   C. splenomegaly is observed in approximately 50% of patients during the second and third week of illness
   D. hepatomegaly and liver tenderness are found in a low percentage of patients as are elevated liver enzymes
   E. generalized lymphadenopathy of gradual onset is characteristic

417. Laboratory findings in infectious mononucleosis are characterized by all of the following, EXCEPT
   A. the height of the heterophil antibody titer is not related to clinical severity of the disease
   B. heterophil antibodies cross-react with other EBV-associated antigens
   C. the heterophil antibody titer in mononucleosis serum is not significantly reduced by guinea-pig kidney absorption but is completely absorbed by beef erythrocytes
   D. during acute mononucleosis there is a marked increase with the total serum IgM
   E. during the first week of illness the WBC may be normal or there may be leukopenia due to granulocytopenia

418. Which of the following does NOT distinguish the infectious mononucleosis caused by EBV from that caused by cytomegalovirus?
   A. Atypical lymphocytosis with fever
   B. Negative heterophil antibodies
   C. Cervical adenopathy
   D. Tonsillar exudate
   E. Sore throat

419. Acute lymphocytosis can be differentiated from infectious mononucleosis due to EBV by all of the following EXCEPT
   A. adenopathy
   B. splenomegaly
   C. atypical lymphocytes
   D. lymphocytosis
   E. heterophil antibodies

420. Of the following viruses, which is LEAST commonly found in lower respiratory illnesses?
   A. Adenovirus
   B. Respiratory syncytial virus
   C. Parainfluenza type 1
   D. Parainfluenza type 3
   E. Parainfluenza type 2

421. The epidemiology and pathology of respiratory syncytial viral infection is characterized by all of the following EXCEPT

    A. it is the most important viral respiratory pathogen of infancy and childhood

    B. its peak incidence occurs in first year of life with most serious illnesses occurring in first six months

    C. maternal serum antibody is protective

    D. evidence that reinfection with RSV frequently triggers wheezing attacks in children with chronic asthma

    E. replication of virus in initial infection occurs in oro- and nasopharynx

422. Clinical features of RVS may be described by all of the following EXCEPT

    A. RSV bronchiolitis usually manifested by wheezing and reaches its peak severity in 48 to 72 hours

    B. CO_2 retention may be presumed to begin when the respiratory rate surpasses 60 per minute

    C. distinction between RSV bronchiolitis and RSV pneumonia is usually easily made

    D. RSV disease in younger infants is generally worse than in older children

    E. RSV pneumonia generally resolves spontaneously in the course of a few weeks

423. Clinical parainfluenza virus is characterized by all of the following EXCEPT

    A. infections are most common in children less than six months of age

    B. it is a frequent cause of infectious croup syndrome

    C. immunity to parainfluenza viruses is incomplete

    D. WBCs average 12,000 to 14,000 with slight predominance of polymorphonuclear granulocytes

    E. the bronchiolitic and pneumonitic syndromes produced by parainfluenza viruses are not clinically different from those caused by RSV

424. The typical adenoviral respiratory infection may be associated with all of the following EXCEPT
    A. pharyngitis
    B. absence of cervical adenitis
    C. conjunctivitis
    D. fever
    E. excretion of virus in feces long after recovery from the illness

425. The clinical picture of rhinoviral disease is characterized by all of the following EXCEPT
    A. it is most commonly associated with upper respiratory disease as compared to lower respiratory disease
    B. there is usually little, if any, fever
    C. there is little tendency to cause pharyngeal exudate
    D. cervical lymphadenopathy is commonly present
    E. secretory antibody appears to be more important than serum antibody in preventing disease

426. The epidemiology and pathogenesis of influenza A viral infection may be characterized by all of the following EXCEPT
    A. major alteration with the surface antigens introduces a new virulent virus into the environment, since antibody against previous antigens will not be protective
    B. the antigenic alteration in influenza virus is an expression of genetic alteration of the viral DNA
    C. antibody to the hemagglutinin (HA) of the virus is apparently more important than antibody to neuraminidase (NA) in controlling infection
    D. new influenza strains may arise by recombination of genetic material from human and animal influenza viruses
    E. course of disease is principally determined by the presence or absence of specific secretory IgA antibody

427. Which of the following does NOT characterize influenza infections?

A. Incubation period is short, usually one to three days

B. Physical and x-ray evidence of pneumonia is generally the rule rather than the exception in influenza illness

C. Localized pneumonia is often caused by secondary infection with pneumococci and *S. aureus*

D. Routine laboratory studies are usually within normal limits with the exception of elevation of ESR

E. Physical findings in the typical case are few

428. Which of the following is NOT characteristic of lymphocytic choriomeningitis?

A. Viral reservoir probably located in house mice

B. Man-to-man transmission

C. Pneumonic symptoms common

D. CSF findings consistent with aseptic meningitis

E. Meningitis is the most important manifestation of the infection in children

429. The pathogenesis and epidemiology of measles are characterized by all of the following EXCEPT

A. although less than 1% of patients develop signs and symptoms of encephalomyelitis, about 50% show EEG changes

B. measles virus has not been recovered from the CSF or CNS tissue of patients with encephalomyelitis

C. single attack confers lifelong immunity

D. the disease is most communicable during the rash stage

E. nearly all patients have demonstrable circulating serum antibodies by the second day of rash

430. Which of the following is FALSE regarding measles immunization?
   A. The attenuated vaccines provide an infection that is communicable
   B. Secondary bacterial infections and neurologic complications that accompany natural or modified measles do not occur following vaccination
   C. Serious complications may occur in children exposed to natural measles after having been vaccinated years before with killed vaccine
   D. Given at the appropriate time, live vaccine provides 95% prophylactic efficacy
   E. It may diminish cutaneous delayed hypersensitivity reaction to tuberculoprotein

431. The epidemiology of mumps (epidemic parotitis) is characterized by all of the following EXCEPT
   A. mumps is endemic at all times
   B. orchitis and meningoencephalitis may occur in the absence of parotitis
   C. transplacental immunity probably accounts for the infrequency of mumps in the first six months after birth
   D. the incubation period may last as long as a month
   E. it is more communicable than measles and varicella

432. The clinical manifestations of mumps are characterized by all of the following EXCEPT
   A. unilateral parotid involvement is more frequent
   B. orchitis is very rare in childhood
   C. submaxillary or sublingual glands may be the only salivary glands involved
   D. meningoencephalitis may be the only evidence of mumps
   E. pancreatitis occurs much less frequently in children than in adults

433. Regarding laboratory tests in patients with mumps, which of the following is FALSE?
    A. WBC is usually within normal limits with a relative lymphocytosis
    B. Elevation of serum or urine amylase is nearly always present in first week of parotitis
    C. A rise in amylase is specific for pancreatitis
    D. Complement fixation is reliable testing for the presence of mumps antibodies
    E. Commercially available mumps skin test antigens should not be used to determine the state of immunity of exposed adults

434. Which of the following does NOT characterize the epidemiology of Coxsackie viral infection?
    A. Group B viruses are associated with epidemic myalgia
    B. Group A viruses are associated with myocarditis and pericarditis
    C. Group A viruses are usually associated with herpangina
    D. Sporadic acute illness with exanthems is associated with groups A and B
    E. Both groups (A and B) are associated with hepatitis

435. Herpangina is manifested by all of the following EXCEPT
    A. it is caused by Coxsackie group A
    B. clinical laboratory findings are normal
    C. lesions are most commonly located on gingiva and buccal mucosa
    D. headache and abdominal symptoms are common
    E. recovery is usually uncomplicated

436. The hand-foot-mouth disease of Coxsackie viral infection is characterized by all of the following EXCEPT
    A. it is caused by Group B virus
    B. constitutional symptoms are usually mild
    C. routine laboratory results are usually within normal limits
    D. skin manifestations include vesicles in mouth, hands, and feet accompanied by a maculopapular rash on extremities
    E. complications are very rare

437. Which of the following disease entities is probably LEAST often associated with ECHO viral infection?
    A. Acute respiratory illness
    B. Diarrhea
    C. Exanthems
    D. Muscle weakness and paralysis
    E. Aseptic meningitis

438. Of the following statements concerning rubella, which is FALSE?
    A. The exanthem is variable and may be scarlatiniform in appearance
    B. It is not as highly contagious as measles
    C. Arthritis is uncommon in children
    D. Thrombocytopenia as a complication is very rare
    E. Adenopathy may persist for weeks

439. Based on reliability, sensitivity, and cost, which of the following tests is most appropriate for clinical use in rubella?
    A. Hemagglutination inhibition (HI)
    B. Complement fixation
    C. Immunofluorescence (IF)
    D. Neutralization
    E. Viral isolation

440. The most common manifestation of congenital rubella in the neonatal period is
    A. congenital heart disease
    B. thrombocytopenic purpura
    C. cataracts
    D. neurologic defects
    E. hepatosplenomegaly

441. Which of the following statements concerning congenital rubella is FALSE?
    A. The risk of fetal abnormalities associated with maternal rubella infection late in the second trimester or later is minimal
    B. The infant may remain chronically infected for months after birth
    C. IgM is the dominant rubella antibody at one year of age
    D. The presence of rubella-specific IgM reflects in utero antibody production by the fetus
    E. Isolation of virus from the blood is rare

442. Which of the following statements concerning trachoma and inclusion conjunctivitis agent (ICA) is FALSE?
   A. Trachoma infection is limited to the eye
   B. Inclusion conjunctivitis agent resides in the genital tract of adults
   C. Conjunctival scarring and corneal vascularization and opacification may occur in trachoma
   D. Infection with inclusion conjunctivitis agent responds poorly to antibodies and may result in corneal scarring
   E. Classified as members of the psittacosis group

443. Of the human rickettsioses, which is NOT associated with a generalized rash?
   A. Epidemic typhus
   B. Rocky Mountain spotted fever
   C. Rickettsial pox
   D. Q fever
   E. Murine typhus

444. From which of the following disease entities does sera NOT agglutinate the proteus antigens used in the Weil-Felix reaction?
   A. Epidemic typhus
   B. Rocky Mountain spotted fever
   C. Rickettsial pox
   D. Scrub typhus
   E. Murine typhus

445. Which of the following statements concerning human rickettsioses is NOT true?
   A. Commonly used antibiotics suppress, but do not destroy, the organisms
   B. Viable pathogenic organisms may be found in lymph nodes of patients convalescing from typhus and Rocky Mountain spotted fever
   C. Weil-Felix reaction is the most reliable test for rickettsial disease
   D. Organisms are highly infective and require intracellular milieu for growth
   E. Pathologic lesion of the exanthamatous rickettsioses includes generalized involvement of small blood vessels

446. Rocky Mountain spotted fever is clinically manifested by all of the following EXCEPT
   A. the exanthem is evidence of vasculitis involving small vessels
   B. CNS involvement is greater in patients with Rocky Mountain spotted fever than in those with other rickettsial diseases
   C. thrombocytopenia is an uncommon finding
   D. the rash usually begins on extremities
   E. CSF is generally normal except for mild lymphocytic pleocytosis

447. Which of the following tests is diagnostic for Rocky Mountain spotted fever?
   A. Proteus OX-19
   B. Proteus OX-2
   C. Complement fixation
   D. Guinea pig inoculation
   E. OX-K

448. Rickettsial pox is characterized by all of the following EXCEPT
   A. presence of an initial lesion that is not painful or pruritic
   B. exanthem is papulovesicular without characteristic distribution
   C. complication and fatalities are rare
   D. elevated proteus OX-19 titers are suggestive of diagnosis
   E. caused by infected mite with *Rickettsia akari*

449. Q fever most often mimics which of the following diseases?
   A. Atypical pneumonia
   B. Varicella
   C. Primary herpetic infection
   D. Rocky Mountain spotted fever
   E. Viral gastroenteritis

IX: Bacterial and Viral Infections
Answers and Comments

337. D. Endotoxic action causes neutrophils to liberate a small protein (leukocyte pyrogen) that acts on anterior hypothalamic nuclei, causing fever. *(REF. 1 — p. 390)*

338. D. Penicillin acts against the bacterial cell wall. *(REF. 1 — p. 398)*

339. A. Penicillin inhibits the transpeptidation reaction and certain other enzymes involved in the structure of peptidoglycan, thus causing sensitive bacteria to produce defective cell walls. *(REF. 1 — p. 398)*

340. B. Aminoglycosides bind irreversibly to individual structural proteins blocking recognition or provoking errors in RNA binding, hence producing the synthesis of faulty protein. *(REF. 1 — p. 399)*

341. A. Sulfonamides are structurally similar to p-aminobenzoic acid and therefore competitively inhibit the enzyme necessary for folic acid metabolism. *(REF. 1 — p. 399)*

342. D. The activity of the aminoglycosides as well as erythromycin is increased in an alkaline medication. *(REF. 1 — p. 400)*

343. B. Activity is increased in acid pH. *(REF. 1 — p. 403)*

344. B. Lincomycin does not penetrate into the CNS. *(REF. 1 — p. 403)*

345. B. Dose-related problems include interference with iron metabolism, decreased circulating reticulocyte count, anemia, and leukopenia. The idiosyncratic reaction of aplastic anemia is not dose-related. *(REF. 1 — p. 406)*

346. B. Group B streptococci along with the slightly less common *E. coli* are currently considered the major organisms. *(REF. 1 — p. 415)*

347. D. Following *H. influenzae, D. pneumoniae* and *N. meningitidis* are the most common. *(REF. 1 — p. 419)*

348. B. Nuchal rigidity is most often absent. *(REF. 1 — p. 418)*

349. B. With the exception of mumps meningoencephalitis CSF sugar is almost always normal. *(REF. 1 — p. 421)*

350. D. The majority of patients in whom an abnormal volume of fluid is obtained have no clinical sign of cerebral damage. *(REF. 1 — p. 425)*

351. C. Several hours to several days may elapse after ingestion of toxin before symptoms appear. *(REF. 1 — p. 428)*

352. C. Prognosis is generally very good; however relapses of clinical illness do occur. *(REF. 1 — p. 430)*

353. D. Nasal diphtheria is seen particularly in infants and very young children and is usually very mild. *(REF. 1 — p. 434)*

354. D. Adenoviral infection of the throat is usually not manifested by pseudomembrane. *(REF. 1 — p. 435)*

355. E. During the phase of bacteremia a migratory polyarthritis is typical. *(REF. 1 — p. 439)*

356. A. Prior infection does not confer immunity. The significance of the immunologic activity is not well understood. *(REF. 1 — p. 438)*

357. D. The pathogenicity of invasive diseases is related not only to the age of the host but also to the presence of type B capsule. *(REF. 1 — p. 443)*

358. B. Most cases of bacteremia are caused by the pneumococcus. *(REF. 1 — p. 444)*

359. C. A raised, warm, tender area that is reddish blue in color is usually found on the cheek. *(REF. 1 — p. 444)*

360. D. A child almost always assumes a sitting position, leaning forward with chin extended. *(REF. 1 — p. 444)*

361. B. Multiple joint involvement is uncommon. *(REF. 1 — p. 444)*

362. C. Meningitis is associated with the second stage of this biphasic disease. *(REF. 1 — p. 448)*

363. A. Although acute meningitis is the most common, fever and rash are other dominant features. *(REF. 1 — p. 450)*

364. E. Adenoviral disease is usually not associated with petechial and maculopopular eruptions. *(REF. 1 — p. 450)*

365. B. Although little experience exists in the use of rifampin in children, it, along with minocycline, is useful in eradicating carriage of meningococci. *(REF. 1 — p. 452)*

366. C. Infiltrate is more reticular (viral-like) and appears to fan from the hilum to the periphery and is usually confined to one lobe. *(REF. 1 — p. 453)*

367. A. RSV infections usually occur in infants and young children, whereas mycoplasmal infection occurs more often in older children and adults. *(REF. 1 — p. 453)*

368. D. Total WBC is usually in the range of 25,000 to 40,000 with a predominance of small mature lymphocytes. These appear in the circulation as a result of the discharge of the marginal pool under influence of lymphocyte promoting factor of *B. pertussis*. *(REF. 1 — p. 456)*

369. D. ECHO viral infection is usually not associated with paroxysmal coughing. *(REF. 1 — p. 457)*

370. A. On cultural growth, there is a late pigment change in colonies that lends a light chocolate hue to those of parapertussis. *(REF. 1 — p. 460)*

371. D. Renal lesions occur late and rarely before five years after infection. *(REF. 1 — p. 464)*

372. D. Nodal involvement with the bronchial wall is common, occurring with a frequency of up to 20%. *(REF. 1 — p. 465)*

373. B. Miliary tuberculosis is an early complication of primary tuberculosis, which occurs usually within the first six weeks of infection and mostly in infants and young children. *(REF. 1 — p. 467)*

374. D. CSF usually demonstrates mild elevation of the WBCs (10 to 350 cells mm^3). *(REF. 1 — p. 469)*

375. B. The most common site is the spine, followed in frequency by the hip and knee with dactylitis of the hands and feet being infrequent complications. *(REF. 1 — p. 469)*

376. B. The other "atypical" organisms are more often associated with pulmonary infection. *(REF. 1 — p. 482)*

377. C. *M. intracellulare* is usually associated with pulmonary disease. *(REF. 1 — p. 482)*

378. D. Lymphadenitis is the most common disease in childhood. *(REF. 1 — p. 482)*

379. A. Most strains are resistant to drug therapy. Excision is the treatment of choice when nodes are easily accessible. *(REF. 1 — p. 483)*

380. A. Ulceroglandular tularemia occurs when organisms gain entry through the skin, which is the most common site of entry. *(REF. 1 — p. 484)*

381. C. Man-to-man transmission has not been reported in tularemia. *(REF. 1 — p. 484)*

382. B. Unlike the skin test for brucella, it does not induce agglutinins in skin-tested individuals. *(REF. 1 — p. 485)*

383. D. Arthritis is the most common localized infection. Osteomyelitis, cystitis, meningitis, endocarditis, and soft tissue abscesses have been reported. *(REF. 1 — p. 488)*

384. D. Typhoid fever is caused by *S. typhi* in all age groups. However, the disease is generally mild in infants, rose spots are rare in infants, and unlike as in older patients, leukocytosis is frequent. Complications are also infrequent in young children. *(REF. 1 — p. 489)*

385. B. Shigella, as a rule, do not invade the bloodstream. *(REF. 1 — p. 491)*

386. A. Leukocytosis is not characteristic of enteropathogenic *E. coli* enteritis. *(REF. 1 — p. 493)*

387. C. Diarrhea does not always accompany staphylococcal food poisoning, but when it does it is relatively mild. *(REF. 1 — p. 497)*

388. E. This is characteristic of all beta-hemolytic streptococci. *(REF. 1 — p. 498)*

389. D. The face is usually spared from rash, with the heaviest concentration in the flexural creases. *(REF. 1 — p. 499)*

390. A. Pneumonia and sepsis are more common in immediate period; meningitis is more common in delayed-onset disease. *(REF. 1 — p. 503)*

391. C. Cardiovascular involvement in childhood disease is rare, contrasted with a 15% incidence, most commonly aortitis, in adults. *(REF. 1 — p. 504)*

392. D. Both antibodies tested in STS and TPI behave similarly. Both disappear from the infant and are unmeasurable in most infants in eight weeks and in all by 12 weeks of age. *(REF. 1 — p. 505)*

393. C. Cat-scratch disease is not transmitted by one human to another. *(REF. 1 — p. 516)*

394. C. Thrombocytopenic purpura, encephalitis, primary atypical pneumonia, and osteomyelitis are unusual clinical manifestations of cat-scratch disease. *(REF. 1 — p. 516)*

395. A. Varicella zoster virus is a member of the herpesvirus group. *(REF. 1 — p. 518)*

396. E. Varicella, like many other viral infections is much more severe in adults than in children. *(REF. 1 — p. 519)*

397. B. The distribution of the lesions is predominantly centripetal. *(REF. 1 — p. 519)*

398. C. The eruption of smallpox is usually centrifugal. *(REF. 1 — p. 520)*

399. D. Clinical manifestations most frequently seen among symptomatic newborns in order of decreasing frequency are hepatosplenomegaly, jaundice, purpura, microcephaly, chorioretinitis, and paraventricular cerebral calcifications. *(REF. 1 — p. 521)*

400. B. If cataracts are associated with a congenital heart lesion the probability of congenital rubella is high. *(REF. 1 — p. 521)*

401. C. Patients with CMV mononucleosis are always heterophil antibody-negative. *(REF. 1 — p. 522)*

402. A. Roseola is characterized by sudden onset of high fever lasting for several days, and with defervescence the rubella-like rash appears. *(REF. 1 — p. 523)*

403. B. Rotavirus is a reo-like virus that rarely causes diarrhea in adults. *(REF. 1 — p. 524)*

404. C. The brown discoloration of urine is often the first clue to the diagnosis of viral hepatitis. *(REF. 1 — p. 525)*

405. B. SGOT and SGPT test for the release of enzymes by damaged hepatic cells. Also useful in the preicteric stage is a test for urine bilirubin. *(REF. 1 — p. 526)*

406. E. Neither serum bilirubin nor SGOT correlate well with the severity of illness, and there is usually no point in determining BSP retention with an icteric patient. *(REF. 1 — p. 526)*

407. B. All others are either outmoded concepts or of undemonstrable value. *(REF. 1 — p. 526)*

408. D. Not only are joint manifestations more common with type B infections but polyarteritis and glomerulonephritis are more common also. *(REF. 1 — p. 529)*

409. D. HB_SAg positivity is an index of carrier state that supervenes in 5% to 10% of overt cases. *(REF. 1 — p. 528)*

410. E. The antigenic and structural integrity are rapidly lost in the presence of intestinal and bacterial enzymes. *(REF. 1 — p. 529)*

411. C. Infectious virus cannot be demonstrated with sensory ganglia; however, by using special cultivation methods of the ganglia, it can be reactivated. *(REF. 1 — p. 532)*

412. B. Neutralizing antibodies are present but do not rise after each recurrence. *(REF. 1 — p. 533)*

413. D. The most common site of involvement is the cervix. *(REF. 1 — p. 535)*

414. B. HSV meningitis is primarily caused by HSV-2, is rarely found in children, but may be encountered in adolescents and in immunologically compromised individuals. *(REF. 1 — p. 535)*

415. D. In lower socioeconomic groups approximately 80% of children have antibody by the age of six years. *(REF. 1 — p. 540)*

416. D. Although hepatomegaly is found in only 10% of patients elevated levels of SGOT and serum LDH are seen in the majority of patients, and these persist for weeks to months after the disease. *(REF. 1 — p. 540)*

417. B. Heterophil antibodies do not cross-react with any known EBV-associated antigens, and the manner in which EBV infection induces these antibodies is not known. *(REF. 1 — p. 541)*

418. A. The characteristics of CMV mononucleosis are atypical lymphocytosis, fever, and hepatosplenomegaly. *(REF. 1 — p. 542)*

419. D. Absolute lymphocytosis is characteristic, but the lymphocytes are small and mature. *(REF. 1 — p. 542)*

420. A. Respiratory syncytial virus and parainfluenza virus types 1, 2, and 3 account for about 70% of all viral isolates. Adenovirus is more often found in URIs. *(REF. 1 — p. 543)*

421. C. Serum maternal antibody provides no protection. It has been postulated that in the absence of secretory antibody, local or systemic cellular immunity, serum antibody may lead to exacerbation of RSV infection. *(REF. 1 — p. 544)*

422. C. Rales and wheezing may be found in both entities so that this distinction is often arbitrary. *(REF. 1 — p. 544)*

423. A. Incidence of infection is highest in the second and third years of life. *(REF. 1 — p. 546)*

424. B. Adenovirus infection usually begins in the pharynx or conjunctivae, and regional lymph nodes are commonly invaded. *(REF. 1 — p. 549)*

425. D. Cervical lymphadenopathy is very uncommon. *(REF. 1 — p. 550)*

426. B. The antigenic alteration in influenza is an expression of genetic alteration of viral RNA. *(REF. 1 — p. 548)*

427. B. Clinical and x-ray evidence of pneumonia is unusual in the uncomplicated case of influenza. *(REF. 1 — p. 548)*

428. C. Pneumonic and bizarre neurologic syndromes have not been reported in children. *(REF. 1 — p. 552)*

429. D. The disease is most communicable during the viremia stage (first seven to ten days after exposure). In addition to being recoverable from the respiratory tract it can also be found in nasopharyngeal secretions, urine, and blood. *(REF. 1 — p. 553)*

430. A. Attenuated vaccines are not associated with communicability. *(REF. 1 — p. 558)*

431. E. Mumps is less communicable than measles, varicella, or pertussis. *(REF. 1 — p. 559)*

432. A. Bilateral involvement occurs with approximately 70% of cases. *(REF. 1 — p. 560)*

433. C. There is some evidence that the increase in amylase is due only to inflammation of parotid glands and that involvement of other than the salivary glands or testes has no effect on amylase levels. *(REF. 1 — p. 561)*

434. A. Group B viruses have most often been associated with cardiac disease. *(REF. 1 — p. 571)*

435. C. Lesions commonly located on the fauces, soft palate, and uvula. *(REF. 1 — p. 571)*

436. A. The hand-foot-mouth disease is caused by Coxsackie virus A5 or A16. *(REF. 1 — p. 571)*

437. B. The association of types 11, 14, and 18 with diarrheal disease has been observed and an etiologic relationship has been suggested. *(REF. 1 — p. 574)*

438. D. Many patients have a slight but definite decrease in platelets during course of uncomplicated rubella, and it usually occurs within 1 week after onset of rash. *(REF. 1 — p. 581)*

439. A. The HI antibody test standardized by the Communicable Disease Center is well suited for general clinical use. The CF test may serve as a useful backup for the HI. *(REF. 1 — p. 581)*

440. B. All of the others occur but may not be manifested until after the neonatal period. *(REF. 1 — p. 585)*

441. C. Except in rare cases, IgG is usually the dominant rubella antibody found in infants at one year of age. *(REF. 1 — p. 585)*

442. D. ICA responds to topical therapy, and although the untreated infection can persist for months, it leaves without residue. *(REF. 1 — p. 594)*

443. D. In Q fever, cutaneous involvement is not apparent, and the disease generally is confined to the lungs and liver. *(REF. 1 — p. 596)*

444. C. Neither the sera from patients with rickettsial pox nor Q fever agglutinate proteus OX-19. *(REF. 1 — p. 598)*

445. C. Specific serologic reactions using rickettsial antigens in complement-fixation, agglutination, or neutralization tests are more reliable. *(REF. 1 — p. 596)*

446. C. Thrombocytopenia is commonly found and is a result of peripheral sequestation or of an injury to the platelets. *(REF. 1 — p. 601)*

447. C. A fourfold rise or higher in complement fixation during the second or third febrile week is diagnostic. *(REF. 1 — p. 601)*

448. D. Proteus OX-19 is not agglutinated by sera of patients with rickettsial pox. *(REF. 1 — p. 602)*

449. A. Respiratory manifestations usually predominate and there is no rash. *(REF. 1 — p. 603)*

X: Mycotic and Parasitic Diseases

DIRECTIONS: Each of the questions or incomplete statements below is followed by five suggested answers or completions. Select the one that is **BEST** in each case.

450. Actinomycosis is characterized by all of the following EXCEPT
   A. it is isolated in nature only from man
   B. it is considered a true fungus
   C. it is responsive to penicillin therapy
   D. aspirated material typically reveals sulfur granules
   E. it produces an indolent granulomatous suppurative infection

451. Infection with *Blastomyces dermatitidis* is characterized by all of the following EXCEPT
   A. the lungs are the primary site of infection
   B. the majority of patients will have positive complement-fixation test
   C. chronic cutaneous blastomycosis is the most common form of North American blastomycosis and is the presenting complaint of most patients
   D. it is responsive to amphotericin B
   E. the pulmonary form is difficult to distinguish from active tuberculosis

452. The clinical picture of coccidioidomycosis may be associated with all of the following EXCEPT
   A. the primary nonfatal form is usually associated with respiratory disease that may be asymptomatic
   B. a negative coccidioidin skin test in a patient with erythema nodosum usually eliminates the possibility of coccidioidomycosis
   C. negative serologic tests virtually rule out the chronic disseminated form of the disease
   D. organisms may be found in sputum, gastric washings, CSF, and pleural or peritoneal fluid
   E. amphotericin B is indicated in primary coccidioidomycosis

453. The primary acute form of histoplasmosis is characterized by all of the following EXCEPT
   A. the primary site is the lungs
   B. it is usually mild and often asymptomatic
   C. a histoplasmin skin test is positive three to five weeks after infection
   D. amphotericin B therapy is indicated
   E. subpleural tubercles are formed

454. The severe disseminated form of histoplasmosis is characterized by all of the following EXCEPT
   A. the skin test is positive in the majority of cases
   B. organisms are frequently obtained from blood, bone marrow aspiration, and lymph node biopsy
   C. it is seen most often in infants and debilitated patients
   D. hepatosplenomegaly and generalized lymphadenophy are commonly seen
   E. lesions of the skin and mucous membranes of the mouth are common in young patients

455. Cryptococcosis is associated with all of the following EXCEPT
   A. it is seen most frequently in patients with serious underlying disease
   B. infection is usually acquired by inhalation
   C. CNS involvement is a rare complication
   D. pulmonary infection may be a common manifestation and may be asymptomatic
   E. its primary source is avian excrement

456. Infection with *Ascaris lumbricoides* is characterized by all of the following EXCEPT
   A. eggs require developmental stage outside the human host
   B. eggs containing the infective second-stage larvae hatch in the soil
   C. intestinal penetration and migration through the liver by larvae are usually of little pathologic importance
   D. the vast majority of ascarids finally settle in the jejunum
   E. Löffler's pneumonia may be a serious manifestation of infection

457. Which of the following signs or symptoms does NOT usually characterize ascariasis?
   A. Urticaria
   B. Cough with hemoptysis
   C. Eosinophilia
   D. Vague abdominal pain
   E. Hepatomegaly

458. Visceral larva migrans is associated with all of the following EXCEPT
   A. humans are not usually the hosts of the dog ascarid, *Toxocara canis*
   B. the larvae migrate most often to the lungs
   C. lesions are necrotizing or granulomatous and heavily infiltrated with eosinophils
   D. the most characteristic clinical picture is of hepatomegaly, eosinophilia, fever, cough, and wheezing
   E. hyperglobulinemia

459. Which of the following is the best definitive diagnostic test for visceral larva migrans?
   A. Liver biopsy
   B. Antihemagglutinin A titer
   C. Serology
   D. Eosinophilia
   E. Bronchoscopy

460. Enterobiasis (*Enterobius vermicularis*) is associated with all of the following EXCEPT
   A. it does not require a host other than the human and does not require soil for maturation
   B. eosinophilia is a common manifestation
   C. ova are infrequently seen in the stool
   D. there is no portal migration
   E. there is no pulmonary migration

461. Hookworm disease (*Necator americanus*) is characterized by all of the following, EXCEPT
   A. migration through the lungs is indispensable to development
   B. a period of time in the soil is necessary for development of larvae
   C. pulmonic infiltrative disease with consolidation is common
   D. a common abnormality is microcytic hypochromic anemia
   E. growth failure may be seen in some patients

462. Amebiasis (*Entamoeba histolytica*) is associated with all of the following EXCEPT
   A. transmission is by ingestion of cysts
   B. trophozoites emerge from cysts as result of the action of digestive enzymes
   C. intestinal bacteria are essential to production of intestinal lesions by trophozoites
   D. intestinal lesions remain superficial
   E. liver abscess is a frequent complication

463. The etiology and epidemiology of toxoplasmosis are characterized by all of the following EXCEPT
   A. toxoplasma is a coccidian parasite of cats
   B. infection may be acquired by ingestion of infective oocysts in the soil or tissue cysts in raw meat
   C. the fetus is at greatest risk from transplacental transmission during the first and second trimester
   D. worldwide distribution is seen
   E. responsible for habitual abortions

464. Which of the following is LEAST often encountered in acute congenital toxoplasmosis seen during the immediate post-natal period?
   A. Intracerebral calcifications
   B. Thrombocytopenic purpura
   C. Severe jaundice
   D. Hepatosplenomegaly
   E. Chorioretinitis

465. Acquired toxoplasmosis is usually associated with all of the following EXCEPT
   A. it is usually asymptomatic
   B. the acute fulminating form with myocarditis and encephalitis is usually fatal in outcome
   C. generalized lymphadenopathy characterizes the sub-acute form
   D. retinochoroiditis is usually seen in the acute fulminant form
   E. its incubation period is unknown

DIRECTIONS: Each set of lettered headings below is followed by a list of numbered words or phrases. For each numbered word or phrase select
   A if the item is associated with (A) *only*,
   B if the item is associated with (B) *only*,
   C if the item is associated with *both* (A) *and* (B),
   D if the item is associated with *neither* (A) *nor* (B).

   A. Blastomycosis
   B. Actinomycosis
   C. Both
   D. Neither

466. Has a pulmonary form of infection

467. Most commonly seen as a chronic cutaneous infection

468. Penicillin is the drug of choice

469. Amphotericin B is the drug of choice

470. Can be seen on microscopic smears of specimens

Directions Summarized			
A	B	C	D
only	only	only	neither
A	B	A,B	A nor B

   A. Histoplasmosis
   B. Cryptococcosis
   C. Both
   D. Neither

471. Infection may be asymptomatic

472. Can cause meningitis even in the nonimmunosuppressed host

473. In systemic disease, amphotericin B is the drug of choice

474. Serologic tests can be helpful in establishing the diagnosis

475. Spread by person-to-person contact

   A. *A. lumbricoides*
   B. *N. americanus*
   C. Both
   D. Neither

476. Migrates through the lungs

477. May cause intestinal obstruction

478. Frequently causes anemia

479. Passes from animal host to man

480. Pyrantel pamoate eradicates infection

   A. *E. histolytica*
   B. *Giardia lamblia*
   C. Both
   D. Neither

481. Creates deep ulcers in colon wall

482. A protozoan

483. Pulmonary migration is a part of life cycle

484. Frequent asymptomatic colonization

485. Can form visceral abscesses

X: Mycotic and Parasitic Diseases
Answers and Comments

450. B. It is a gram-positive, anaerobic, branching filamentous actinomycetes bacterium. *(REF. 1 — p. 609)*

451. B. Apparently less than 50% of the sera from patients with proved blastomycosis gives a positive complement-fixation test. Furthermore, since cross-reaction between North American blastomycosis and histoplasmosis is not uncommon, a single serologic examination must be interpreted with caution. *(REF. 1 — p. 611)*

452. E. The primary form of the disease usually requires no therapy, since it is self-limited. Intravenous amphotericin B is indicated in the disseminated form. *(REF. 1 — p. 613)*

453. D. In the usual mild self-limited attacks no specific antifungal therapy is indicated. *(REF. 1 — p. 616)*

454. A. The skin test may remain negative in about 50% of cases, although the complement-fixation test usually, if not always, turns positive. *(REF. 1 — p. 616)*

455. C. CNS infection is a common manifestation, and meningitis is regarded as the most frequent cause of mycotic meningitis. *(REF. 1 — p. 617)*

456. B. Larvae never hatch in the soil but require oral ingestion and the action of enzymes in the duodenum to break through the egg shell. *(REF. 1 — p. 621)*

457. E. Migration through the portal system and liver usually does not cause significant pathology. *(REF. 1 — p. 625)*

458. B. Migration is usually to the liver, less frequently to lungs, kidneys, heart, brain, eye, and striated muscle. *(REF. 1 — p. 626)*

459. A. All other examinations are nonspecific. *(REF. 1 — p. 626)*

460. B. Eosinophilia is seldom observed in enterobiasis. *(REF. 1 — p. 627)*

461. C. Pulmonary consolidation during lung phase is distinctly uncommon. *(REF. 1 — p. 629)*

462. D. In severe infections the colonic ulcers may extend to the peritoneal surface with perforation. *(REF. 1 — p. 646)*

463. E. Transmission to the fetus occurs only if the primary infection occurs during pregnancy. Responsibility for habitual abortion is no longer regarded as valid. *(REF. 1 — p. 662)*

464. A. Intracerebral calcification is usually found in the subacute form and is not observed until sometime after birth. *(REF. 1 — p. 663)*

465. D. Retinochoroiditis is usually a self-limited disease but occasionally may become progressive and threaten vision. *(REF. 1 — p. 664)*

466. C. Actinomycosis and blastomycosis can appear as primarily
467. A. pulmonary infections. The diagnosis can be suggested by
468. B. examination of smears of material from the lesions. Peni-
469. A. cillin is the drug of choice for actinomycosis, while ampho-
470. C. tericin B is used in blastomycosis. Blastomycosis most
commonly appears as a chronic cutaneous infection, while actinomycosis does not. *(REF. 1 — pp. 609, 611)*

471. C. Histoplasmosis and cryptococcosis can be present in the
472. B. lungs of asymptomatic hosts. Serology is helpful in the
473. C. diagnosis of both disorders. The drug of choice in the
474. C. systemic diseases created by these organisms is ampho-
475. D. tericin B. Cryptococcosis is renowned for its propensity for
the CNS while histoplasma is not. Neither of these disorders is spread by person-to-person contact. *(REF. 1 — p. 616)*

476. C. Ascaris and necator are roundworm infections that have
477. A. pulmonary migration as part of their life cycle, but neither
478. B. is transmitted from animals to man. Necator can cause
479. D. blood loss anemia while ascaris has been known to cause
480. C. obstruction of ducts and intestines. Both parasites can be
eradicated with pyrantel pamoate. *(REF. 1 — pp. 621-628)*

481. A. Entamoeba can be a very invasive organism, causing deep
482. C. colonic ulcers and abscesses in many organs including the

483. D. brain and liver. It can be found in symptomless carriers
484. C. and it does not have a pulmonary migration. Giardia is
485. A. also a protozoan but is of low virulence and does not form
abscess. It also can be found in asymptomatic carriers, but
it lives mainly in the small bowel and not the colon. Like entamoeba
it does not exhibit pulmonary migration. *(REF. 2 — pp. 1015-1017)*

XI: Endocrine and Metabolic Disorders

DIRECTIONS: Each of the questions or incomplete statements below is followed by five suggested answers or completions. Select the **one** that is **BEST** in each case.

---

486. Phenylketonuria (PKU) is a metabolic disorder in which
    A. melanocytes cannot form melanin
    B. phenylalanine cannot be converted to tyrosine
    C. histidine cannot be converted to urocanic acid
    D. valine cannot be deaminated
    E. methylmalonyl-CoA cannot be metabolized

487. All of the following are characteristic of maple syrup urine disease EXCEPT
    A. infants appear well at birth
    B. early manifestations include feeding difficulty, irregular respirations, or loss of Moro reflex
    C. convulsions are a rare complication
    D. symptoms begin three to five days after birth
    E. the disease is caused by branched-chain ketoaciduria

488. Propionic acidemia is characterized by all of the following EXCEPT
    A. it is a disorder of branched-chain amino acid
    B. elevated concentrations of propionate in body fluids
    C. recurrent episodes of metabolic acidosis and massive ketosis
    D. neutropenia, thrombocytopenia, and osteoporosis
    E. a dramatic response to relatively high doses of cortisone

489. Homocystinuria is characterized by all of the following EXCEPT
    A. it is the most common inherited disorder of amino acid metabolism
    B. the disorder involves the sulfur-containing amino acids
    C. most patients are mentally retarded
    D. death usually occurs before age one year
    E. spontaneous arterial and venous thromboembolic phenomena are prominent

490. Which of the following represents a disorder of amino acid transport?
    A. Phenylketonuria
    B. Tyrosinosis
    C. Alkaptonuria
    D. Homocystinuria
    E. Hartnup disease

491. All of the following are characteristic of Lesch-Nyhan syndrome EXCEPT
    A. severe mental retardation
    B. cerebral palsy
    C. choreoathetosis
    D. self-destructive biting
    E. renal aminoglycinuria

492. All of the following are correct statements regarding galactosemia EXCEPT
    A. it is inherited as an autosomal recessive disorder
    B. the infant usually appears normal at birth, and the clinical signs appear after initiation of milk feedings
    C. hepatomegaly is a late sign
    D. lethargy and hypotonia are frequent findings
    E. the signs may resemble sepsis

493. Hereditary fructose intolerance is characterized by all of the following EXCEPT
    A. symptomatology when fructose is ingested in diet
    B. hypoglycemia, tremors, disorientation are present
    C. chronic ingestion resembles galactosemia
    D. enzyme defect – deficiency of hepatic aldolase
    E. treatment involves using cortisone because of its gluconeogenic effect

494. The most common hereditable lipid disease is
A. Gaucher's disease
B. metachromatic leukodystrophy
C. Niemann-Pick disease
D. Tay-Sachs disease
E. Fabry's disease

495. All of the following are anticipated on the administration of growth hormone to hypopituitary dwarfs EXCEPT
A. rapid growth of the skeletal system
B. disproportionate increase in skeletal maturation
C. calcium retention
D. fall in serum urea
E. mobilization from fat of free fatty acids

496. All of the following are characteristic of idiopathic hypopituitarism EXCEPT
A. it is probably more common than hypopituitarism of organic origin
B. the chief complaint is usually short stature
C. it is believed to have a hypothalamic origin
D. diabetes insipidus does not occur with this disorder
E. carbohydrate function studies are normal in patients with STH deficiency

497. In the diagnostic evaluation of a child with short stature psychosocial dwarfism is being considered. Which of the following is NOT associated with this disorder?
A. Psychologically disturbed child with emotional deprivation
B. Short stature, polyphagia, polydipsia, and polyuria
C. Shyness and temper tantrums
D. Delayed skeletal development
E. Diagnosis proved by dramatic response to growth hormone

498. Hyperpituitarism may present as a problem of overgrowth. All of the following have been associated with hyperpituitarism EXCEPT
    A. headaches are common
    B. prognathism and widening of spaces between the teeth
    C. elevated serum phosphorus level
    D. bone age is normal or minimally advanced
    E. accelerated sexual development and precocious sexual functioning

499. The blood ADH level is high in all of the following EXCEPT
    A. nephrotic syndrome
    B. pain and after anesthesia
    C. after cardiac surgery
    D. the use of most pain medications
    E. cirrhosis

500. All of the following are characteristic of congenital adrenal hyperplasia EXCEPT
    A. deficient production of cortisol starts about two weeks after birth
    B. excessive secretion of adrenal androgens in the female fetus causes masculinization of the external genitalia
    C. acute adrenal crisis of salt-losing form is due to absence of secretion of aldosterone
    D. infants have poor appetites and fail to gain weight
    E. excessive loss of sodium results in severe water loss and dehydration

501. Which of the following is NOT characteristic of adrenogenital syndrome?
    A. Hypersecretion of adrenal androgens causes symptoms of virilism and increased protein anabolism
    B. Virilizing adrenal tumors are rarely palpable but can displace kidney from its normal position
    C. Urinary 17-ketosteroids are decreased
    D. Virilizing adrenal tumors do not produce excessive amounts of cortisol
    E. In boys and girls muscles are well developed

502. All of the following are characteristic of congenital hypothyroidism EXCEPT
   A. infants are born with little or no evidence of thyroid hormone deficiency
   B. classic facies is a result of accumulation of myxedema in subcutaneous tissues and tongue
   C. prolonged hypothyroidism results in muscular hypotonia and mental deficits
   D. T4 values are low and thyroid-stimulating hormone (TSH) concentrations are high in newborns
   E. the best guide to measure effectiveness of therapy is to observe physical changes

503. The presence of a goiter at birth is usually a result of
   A. ingestion of goitrogenic substances by the mother
   B. congenital hypothyroidism
   C. severe peroxidase deficiencies
   D. thyroglossal duct abnormalities
   E. thyroiditis congenita

504. All of the following are characteristic of juvenile thyrotoxicosis EXCEPT
   A. it occurs almost exclusively as a consequence of hyperfunctioning nodules
   B. onset is insidious with increasing nervousness, palpitations, and increased appetite
   C. rarely do children show a weight increase with onset of disease
   D. behavior abnormalities and declining school performance are prominent
   E. signs and symptoms are similar to those produced by a hyperactive sympathetic nervous system

505. Female pseudohermaphroditism is associated with all of the following EXCEPT
   A. presence of ovaries, female ducts, and varying degrees of masculine differentiation of the urogenital sinus and external genitalia
   B. a positive sex chromatin pattern
   C. congenital virilizing adrenal hyperplasia
   D. a relative increase in hydrocortisone production
   E. increased secretion of ACTH

506. All of the following represent inborn errors in the metabolism of tyrosine EXCEPT

A. albinism

B. alkaptonuria

C. parkinsonism

D. Chédiak-Steinbrinck-Higashi syndrome

E. PKU

507. The parent of a three-month-old reports that "His diapers turn black when they dry out." You perform a urine test and determine that the urine has reducing properties, and that it has a positive reaction to Benedict's reagent. The most likely diagnosis is

A. methioninemia

B. alkaptonuria

C. tyrosinemia

D. phenylketonuria

E. vitamin A deficiency

508. Children with latent diabetes (chemical diabetes)

A. are really not asymptomatic but have undetected clinical signs

B. have an abnormal fasting blood glucose concentration

C. have a postprandial blood sugar that is hyperglycemic

D. exhibit a normal glucose tolerance curve

E. have a disease of no clinical significance

509. The classic clinical features of diabetes mellitus in a child consist of

A. polyuria, polydipsia, polyphagia, and weight loss

B. polyuria, enuresis, dysphagia, and stable weight

C. polyphagia, diarrhea, enuresis, and emesis

D. polyuria, tremors, blurred vision, and flank pain

E. polyuria, headache, nausea, and convulsions

510. Nesidioblastosis refers to

A. pulmonary infarction and hemosiderosis

B. thyroiditis secondary to blastomycosis

C. beta-cell hyperplasia of the pancreas

D. granuloma of the ovary

E. alpha-cell tumor of the pituitary

511. Increased secretion of insulin in response to leucine has been associated with all of the following EXCEPT
    A. Prader-Willi syndrome
    B. Laurence-Moon-Biedl syndrome
    C. lipodystrophy
    D. Beckwith syndrome
    E. chlorpropamide pretreatment of normal individuals

512. The most common cause of hypoglycemia in childhood is
    A. diabetes mellitus
    B. ketotic hypoglycemia
    C. leucine sensitivity
    D. beta-cell adenoma
    E. glucose-6-phosphate deficiency

513. Pathognomonic signs of hypoglycemia in a five-year-old are
    A. sweating, pallor, and fatigue
    B. pallor, tremors, and nervousness
    C. bradycardia, nervousness, and fever
    D. drowsiness, eye-rolling, and sweating
    E. none of the above

514. All of the following are characteristic of growth hormone of the anterior lobe of the pituitary gland EXCEPT
    A. GH is a protein with 188 amino acids
    B. the hormone is species-specific; only primate growth hormone is effective in man
    C. deficiency of growth hormone results in dwarfism and an excess causes gigantism or acromegaly
    D. growth hormone stimulates skeletal and protein anabolism by the production of intermediary hormones called somatomedins
    E. growth hormone levels remain consistent throughout the day; random samples fail to reveal deficiencies

515. Relatively common causes of diabetes insipidus include all of the following EXCEPT
    A. tumors of suprasellar and chiasmatic regions, particularly craniopharyngiomas
    B. reticuloendothelioses
    C. encephalitis, sarcoidosis, leukemia
    D. genetic faults
    E. operative procedures in the pituitary or hypothalamic regions

---

DIRECTIONS: Each group of questions below consists of five lettered headings followed by a list of numbered words, phrases or statements. For **each** numbered word, phrase or statement, select the **one** lettered heading that is most closely associated with it. Each lettered heading may be selected once, more than once, or not at all.

A. Phenylketonuria
B. Isovaleric acidemia
C. Alkaptonuria
D. Hartnup disease
E. Propionic acidemia

516. Mental and physical retardation, osteoporosis, and periodic thrombocytopenia

517. Associated with the odor of "sweaty feet"

518. Arthritis and ochronosis

519. Caused by the absence of the hepatic enzyme phenylalanine hydroxylase

520. Defect in the transport of tryptophan by the intestinal mucosa and renal tubule

521. High frequency among fair-skinned, blue-eyed blondes with this disorder

A. Galactosemia
B. Lactase deficiency
C. von Gierke's disease (glycogenosis type I)
D. McArdle syndrome (glycogenosis type V)
E. Pompe's disease (glycogenosis type II)

522. Found mainly in Orientals and Africans

523. Caused by decreased glucose-6-phosphatase activity

524. Primarily myocardial deposition of carbohydrate

525. Caused by decreased phosphorylase activity in striated muscle

526. Patients frequently have cataracts

527. Refractory hypoglycemia is frequent

    A. Gaucher's disease
    B. Hunter's syndrome
    C. Tay-Sachs disease
    D. Acute intermittent porphyria
    E. Hurler's syndrome

528. Seen exclusively in males

529. Very high incidence in persons with Ashkenazi Jewish ancestry

530. Associated with cataracts

531. An abnormality in heme metabolism

532. Caused by β-glucosidase deficiency

533. Caused by N-acetylgalactosaminidase

    A. Congenital adrenal hyperplasia
    B. Cushing's syndrome
    C. Diabetes insipidus
    D. Hyperthyroidism
    E. Hyperaldosteronism

534. Causes hypernatremia

535. Seen in Bartter's syndrome

536. May be virilizing in the female

537. Associated with abnormally elevated cortisol secretion

538. Associated with an abnormal circulating gamma globulin

539. May be associated with sodium wasting

XI: Endocrine and Metabolic Disorders Answers and Comments

486. B. As a result of the inability to convert phenylalanine to tyrosine there is an accumulation of phenylpyruvic acid, which is excreted in the urine. In classic PKU the major clinical problem is mental retardation. The fundamental biochemical defect in PKU is the absence of phenylalanine hydroxylase. *(REF. 1 — p. 673)*

487. C. Convulsions are characteristic of the disease. The infant develops opisthotonos and generalized muscular rigidity. Signs of decerebrate rigidity are seen prior to death, which occur within two to four weeks. *(REF. 1 — p. 679)*

488. E. The management of these patients is directed toward diets in which very small amounts of protein are supplemented with amino acids other than offending ones: isoleucine, methionine, valine, and threonine. *(REF. 1 — p. 680)*

489. A. Homocystinuria is the second most common inherited disorder of amino acid metabolism. In this regard, phenylketonuria occurs with greater frequency. *(REF. 1 — p. 684)*

490. E. Hartnup disease is a disorder in which the transport of some amino acids (e.g., tryptophan) is abnormal in the intestine and in the renal tubule. *(REF. 1 — p. 689)*

491. E. The metabolic deficit in Lesch-Nyhan syndrome is hyperuricemia. Children with this disorder may excrete over 600 mg/day of uric acid. The disease is transmitted as an X-linked recessive, involving the activity of the enzyme hypoxanthine guanine phosphoribosyl transferase. *(REF. 1 — p. 691)*

492. C. In galactosemia there is early evidence of liver involvement. Hepatomegaly is a common and constant finding. Jaundice is frequent and death may occur early from hepatic failure. *(REF. 1 — pp. 713–714)*

493. E. Treatment of hereditary fructose intolerance includes control of 1) IV administration of glucose-containing fluids for the acute symptoms and 2) avoidance of fructose- and sucrose-containing foods for the long term. *(REF. 1 — pp. 715–716)*

494. D. Tay-Sachs disease occurs in persons of Ashkenazi Jewish ancestry; gene frequency is one in 60 persons. The incidence is much less frequent in offspring of non-Jewish ancestry. The disorder is the result of the absence of N-acetylgalactosaminidase. *(REF. 1 — p. 748)*

495. B. Unlike the response to testosterone treatment, rapid growth of the skeletal system with administration of growth hormone is not accompanied by a proportionate increase in skeletal maturation. *(REF. 1 — pp. 1603–1604)*

496. E. Carbohydrate function studies have been reported to be abnormal in about 65% of patients with STH deficiency. Many of the patients have hypoglycemia at the fourth or fifth hour of an oral glucose tolerance test. *(REF. 1 — pp. 1608–1609)*

497. E. The diagnosis of psychosocial dwarfism can only be proved by removing the child from his noxious environment and observing more rapid growth in a favorable environment. Rapid growth spurts are reported when these children are relocated in a more advantageous environment. *(REF. 1 — pp. 1611–1612)*

498. E. The onset of sexual development is either normal or late. Sexual maturation proceeds slowly, and hypogonadism ultimately occurs. *(REF. 1 — p. 1612)*

499. D. ADH blood levels are increased in all hyponatremic states. Blood ADH is high in shock, nephrotic syndrome, cirrhosis, pain, after surgical procedures, and diseases characterized by hypoproteinemia and edema. ADH levels are increased following the administration of vincristine. *(REF. 1 — p. 1618)*

500. A. Congenital adrenal hyperplasia is, as the name states, a congenital disease. The deficiency of production of cortisol starts during fetal life. *(REF. 1 — p. 1633)*

501. C. Urinary neutral 17-ketosteroids are usually greatly elevated. The elevation is due in part to the increase in dehydroepiandrosterone (DHA), which represents 50% or more of the total urinary 17-KS. Virilizing adrenal tumors show no suppression of plasma androgen urinary 17-KS during two dexamethasone suppression tests. *(REF. 1 — pp. 1646, 1647)*

502. E. The best guide to measure success of therapy is to monitor the circulating levels of T₄ and TSH. History and physical examination are important, but they may not reveal mild hypothyroidism or hyperthyroidism. *(REF. 1 — pp. 1675–1676)*

503. A. In the U.S., the most common cause of neonatal goiter is the maternal ingestion of large doses of iodides during pregnancy. The iodides are usually found in expectorants (prescribed for asthma) or for treatment of maternal thyrotoxicosis. Other goitrogens include: thioureas, sulfonamides, and hematinic medications containing cobalt. *(REF. 1 — p. 1679)*

504. A. Juvenile thyrotoxicosis (Graves' disease) occurs almost exclusively as a result of diffuse thyroid hyperplasia rather than hyperfunctioning nodules. Girls are affected six times more frequently than boys, and there is a sharp increase in the disease during early adolescence. *(REF. 1 — pp. 1684–1685)*

505. D. The disorder is caused by an inborn error of adrenocortical biosynthesis that results in relative deficiency of hydrocortisone production, increased secretion of ACTH, and relative excess of androgenic hormones and other steroids. The most common cause is congenital virilizing adrenal hyperplasia, accounting for approximately 50% of all patients with ambiguous external genitalia. *(REF. 1 — p. 1697)*

506. E. PKU is a defect in amino acid metabolism involving phenylalanine. There is an absence of activity of the hepatic enzyme, phenylalanine hydroxylase. As a result, the conversion of phenylalanine to tyrosine is impaired with a resultant accumulation of phenylalanine. In untreated neonates, the level of phenylalanine may reach 60 to 80 mg/dl. *(REF. 2 — pp. 492–496)*

507. B. Alkaptonuria is the most likely diagnosis. The defect is a disorder of phenylalanine-tyrosine metabolism. There is an accumulation in the body and an excretion in the urine of homogentisic acid. The "black diaper" is caused by the oxidation and polymerization of the homogentisic acid. *(REF. 2 — p. 501)*

508. C. Chemical diabetes is associated with no symptoms, normal fasting blood glucose, postprandial hyperglycemia, and an abnormal glucose tolerance test. Approximately 15% to 35% of siblings of diabetic children (requiring insulin) have chemical diabetes. However, only 3% to 9% develop overt diabetes. The difference suggests that chemical diabetes is a relatively stable condition. *(REF. 2 — p. 1584)*

509. A. Polyuria, polyphagia, polydipsia, and weight loss are physiologically related to the inability to synthesize and produce insulin in response to food ingestion. The deficit may occur gradually and reflects the rate of decline in response to beta-cell stimulation. *(REF. 2 — p. 1586)*

510. C. Beta-cell hyperplasia, or nesidioblastosis, causes hypoglycemia. The cause for the islet cell hyperplasia is unknown. It has been reported as a familial disorder associated with multiple endocrine adenomatosis. *(REF. 2 — pp. 1600–1601)*

511. D. In the conditions cited, hypersecretion of insulin occurs in response to glucose, and in addition may be leucine-sensitive. Beckwith syndrome is associated with hyperplasia of the pancreatic islets. Hypoglycemia occurs in the first few days of life and disappears spontaneously. *(REF. 2 — p. 1601)*

512. B. Ketotic hypoglycemia accounts for more than 50% of cases of hypoglycemia in childhood. The usual age of onset is between 18 months and five years. There is generally a spontaneous remission. Males are affected more frequently than females. The attacks respond to glucose administration. *(REF. 2 — p. 1603)*

513. E. There are no pathognomonic signs of hypoglycemia in children. The signs are very mercurial and differ from child to child. The child may exhibit variations of sweating, pallor, fatigue, tachycardia, and nervousness caused by an excessive secretion of epinephrine. CNS signs include headache, irritability, behavioral changes, confusion, seizures, and coma. *(REF. 2 — p. 1606)*

514. E. Random levels of growth hormone are erratic. A short period of exercise enough to make the child breathless can cause a stimulation of production of growth hormone. After age three to six months, a definite cycle is established with sharp rises of growth hormone levels during sleep. *(REF. 2 — pp. 1611–1612)*

515. D. Diabetes insipidus results from the lack of the antidiuretic hormone arginine vasopressin. Any lesion that damages the neurohypophysial unit may result in diabetes insipidus. Tumors and in-filtrative disorders can do this, as well as basal skull fractures. Only in a minority of instances is the condition due to heredity. Autosomal dominant and X-linked recessive inheritance is known. *(REF. 2 — p. 1618)*

516. E. Phenylketonuria is caused by the absence of the hepatic
517. B. enzyme phenylalanine hydroxylase and the frequency is
518. C. high among fair-skinned and blue-eyed persons. Patients
519. A. with isovaleric acidemia are said to have the odor of
520. D. "sweaty feet" because of the accumulation of short-
521. A. chained fatty acids. Hartnup disease is caused by a defect
in the transport of tryptophan in the intestinal mucosa and renal tubule. Infants with propionic acidemia frequently present with mental and physical retardation, osteoporosis, and periodic thrombocytopenia. Alkaptonuria is characterized by the accumulation and excretion in the urine of homogentisic acid and its oxidation products. The slow accumulation of the black polymer of homogentisic acid in cartilage produces a black discoloration: alkaptonuric ochronosis. *(REF. 2 — pp. 496–508)*

522. B. Von Gierke's disease, caused by glucose-6-phosphatase
523. C. deficiency is associated with severe refractory hypo-
524. E. glycemia. Galactosemia also can cause hypoglycemia
525. D. (along with cataracts), but it responds dramatically to
526. A. treatment. McArdle syndrome is caused by decreased
527. C. phosphorylase activity in striated muscle. Pompe's dis-
ease causes deposition of carbohydrate in the myo-cardium. Lactase deficiency is seen primarily in people of Oriental or African ancestry. *(REF. 2 — pp. 521–540, 1080)*

528. B. Tay-Sachs disease is caused by N-acetylgalactosa-
529. C. minidase deficiency and is of very high incidence among
530. E. persons of Ashkenazi Jewish ancestry. Hunter's
531. D. syndrome is an X-linked recessive disorder and is thus seen
532. A. only in males and is not associated with cataracts, while
533. C. patients with Hurler's syndrome have cataracts. Gaucher's
disease is caused by a beta-glucosidase deficiency. Acute intermittent porphyria is caused by a defect in heme metabolism. *(REF. 1 — pp. 747–759)*

534. C. Congenital adrenal hyperplasia may be virilizing in the
535. E. female and may be associated with sodium wasting (alpha-
536. A. hydroxylase deficiency). Cushing's syndrome is associated

537. B. with an abnormally high secretion of cortisol. Hyperaldo-
538. D. steronism is seen as a feature of Bartter's syndrome.
539. A. Hypernatremia is seen in diabetes insipidus. Long-acting
thyroid stimulator is a 75 gamma globulin found in many
patients with hyperthyroidism. *(REF. 1 — p. 1599)*

XII: Circulatory System

DIRECTIONS: Each of the questions or incomplete statements below is followed by five suggested answers or completions. Select the one that is BEST in each case.

540. The anatomic closure of the foramen ovale takes place at about
    A. 24 hours
    B. three to five days
    C. 14 to 21 days
    D. four months
    E. 12 months

541. Percussion of the heart borders may be useful in the diagnosis of all of the following EXCEPT
    A. pericardial effusion
    B. dextrocardia
    C. pneumothorax
    D. lobar atelectasis
    E. bronchopneumonia

542. All of the following statements concerning the auscultation of heart sounds in children are true EXCEPT
    A. a third heart sound is common in normal children
    B. the second heart sound is due to closure of the semilunar valves
    C. the first heart sound is reduced in intensity when cardiac output is increased
    D. a fourth heart sound is generally associated with significant obstruction to ventricular ejection
    E. the origin of the normal first heart sound is debatable

543. Which of the following statements regarding innocent heart murmurs is FALSE?
    A. Thirty percent of children at a single random auscultation may have this murmur
    B. Loudness of murmur may be variable from exam to exam
    C. Patients will have normal ECGs and x-ray films
    D. Murmurs of this variety increase with the Valsalva maneuver
    E. They are unrelated to cardiac disturbance or anatomic abnormality

544. Which of the following characteristics most clearly differentiates the venous hum from patent ductus arteriosus?
    A. Position of auscultation on the chest wall
    B. Heard in both systole and diastole
    C. Venous hum murmur is always of low intensity
    D. Exaggeration or disappearance of murmur by position of head
    E. Changes in intensity with exercise

545. In which of the following situations is further clinical evaluation indicated?
    A. A newborn with heart rate of 130
    B. A two-year-old with heart rate of 110
    C. A newborn with pulse rate of 90 during sleep
    D. A two-month-old infant with pulse rate of 130
    E. A crying newborn with pulse rate of 260

546. Which of the following statements concerning the determination of arterial blood pressure is true?
    A. With cuff technique blood pressure is normally lower in the leg than arm
    B. Flush blood pressure is equal to diastolic pressure
    C. Blood pressure varies little with the age of child until the late teens
    D. Exercise or excitement may raise systolic pressure of children as much as 40 to 50 mm Hg above usual levels
    E. Use of a cuff that is too large will result in false high blood pressure readings

547. Which of the following statements concerning roentgeno-graphic exam of the heart is FALSE?
   A. X-rays taken six feet from patient represent fairly accu-rately the size of heart and chest
   B. When cardiac width is 7 1/2 times that of maximal chest width, the heart is usually enlarged
   C. The transverse diameter of the heart is approximately 3% to 4% of body height
   D. The cardiac shadow width is increased on x-rays made on expiration
   E. Lordotic views are unacceptable for evaluation of heart size

548. Significant differences between neonatal circulation and that of older infants include all of the following EXCEPT
   A. right-to-left shunting through foramen ovale
   B. neonate's pulmonary vasculature retains ability to con-strict in response to hypoxemia
   C. muscular mass of right ventricle equals that of left
   D. some blood flow may occur through the ductus for the first few days after birth
   E. newborn infants have a relatively low oxygen consump-tion at rest

549. All of the following statements concerning fetal circulation are true EXCEPT
   A. blood flow through umbilical vein averages 175 ml/kg and pressure of approximately 12 mm Hg
   B. O_2 saturation is almost 100%
   C. pO_2 is 30 mm Hg
   D. approximately one-half of umbilical venous blood by-passes the liver
   E. the cerebral arteries' blood pO_2 is higher than that of the femoral arteries

550. The incidence of cardiovascular malformations at birth is
   A. eight per 1,000
   B. 15 per 1,000
   C. five per 1,000
   D. 20 per 1,000
   E. one per 1,000

551. Cardiovascular malformations account for what percentage of deaths caused by congenital defects in first year of life?
    A. 25%
    B. 50%
    C. 75%
    D. 10%
    E. 35%

552. The cardiac defect associated with maternal and fetal rubella infection is
    A. aortic valvular insufficiency
    B. pulmonic valve insufficiency
    C. patent ductus arteriosus
    D. mitral valve insufficiency
    E. dextrocardia and pulmonic stenosis

553. Etiologic factors associated with congenital heart disease include all of the following EXCEPT
    A. maternal viral infections
    B. radiation during pregnancy
    C. maternal diabetes
    D. maternal drug ingestion
    E. psychotic illness in the mother

554. Family studies of the incidence of congenital heart disease show all of the following EXCEPT
    A. incidence in liveborn siblings of probands is between 14 to 22 per 1,000
    B. incidence of congenital heart disease in parents is low
    C. pulmonary stenosis has the highest incidence of all lesions in siblings
    D. concordance of the lesions in siblings varies from 35 to 56%
    E. generally both infants of a twin birth will exhibit a congenital heart lesion

555. Chromosomal abnormalities commonly associated with congenital heart defects include all of the following EXCEPT
    A. Down's syndrome
    B. trisomy E
    C. Turner's syndrome
    D. Klinefelter's syndrome
    E. trisomy D

556. Tetralogy of Fallot is classified as a congenital heart lesion with patients exhibiting all of the following EXCEPT
    A. cyanosis
    B. ventricle or septal defect
    C. right ventricular hypertrophy
    D. obstruction to right ventricular outflow
    E. aortic stenosis

557. All of the following are characteristic of cyanosis in the patient with tetralogy of Fallot EXCEPT
    A. it is most prominent in mucous membranes of lips and mouth
    B. it will give skin surface a dusky color
    C. it is always present at birth
    D. it can be relieved somewhat by increased FIO2
    E. it may give the sclerae a gray discoloration

558. In the management of paroxysmal dyspneic attacks in patients with tetralogy of Fallot, all of the following pertain EXCEPT
    A. attacks are preventable by avoidance of excitement and exercise
    B. knee-chest position may give relief
    C. O_2 administration may alleviate symptoms
    D. propranolol has been used successfully in some patients
    E. attacks are most prominent during the first two years of life

559. Complications in patients with tetralogy of Fallot include all of the following EXCEPT
    A. cerebral thrombosis
    B. brain abscess
    C. bacterial endocarditis, common in unoperated patients
    D. bleeding tendencies
    E. congestive heart failure which may be precipitated by iron deficiency anemia

560. Which of the following is true concerning transposition of the great arteries?
    A. Condition is rare as a cause of death in the first year of life in patients with cyanotic heart disease
    B. Defects of ventricular system are rare
    C. Polycythemia is usual in older infants
    D. Condition occurs predominantly in females
    E. Marked increase in pulmonary vascular resistance is common in neonates

561. The emergency surgical procedure for hypoxic patients with transposition of the great arteries seeks to establish all of the following EXCEPT
    A. a large interatrial shunt
    B. reduction of left atrial pressure
    C. relief of tachypnea
    D. an increase in arterial oxygen saturation
    E. repair of small ventricular septal defect

562. In the neonate with isolated transposition of the great arteries all of the following are true EXCEPT
    A. recognition of cyanosis may be delayed in the first few days of life
    B. normal birthweight
    C. murmurs are absent in the majority in the first few days of life
    D. tachypnea is present
    E. massive cardiomegaly is common

563. The patient with transposition of the great arteries with a large ventricular septal defect has
    A. a good prognosis
    B. no response to atrial septostomy
    C. dominant clinical findings of congestive heart failure
    D. obvious cyanosis within the first few hours of life
    E. a better prognosis than the patient with small ventricular septal defect and transposition of the great arteries

564. Patients with Ebsteins's disease have all of the following characteristics EXCEPT
  A. downward displacement of an abnormal tricuspid valve into right ventricle
  B. may have no symptoms until adulthood
  C. both systolic and diastolic murmur
  D. small right atrium and enormous right ventricle
  E. large, sail-like anterior tricuspid leaflet

565. Hypoplastic left heart syndrome may be accompanied by all of the following symptoms EXCEPT
  A. dyspnea
  B. hepatomegaly
  C. cyanosis
  D. femoral pulses increased and brachial pulses decreased
  E. metabolic acidosis

566. In cases of hypoplastic left heart, x-rays demonstrate all of the following EXCEPT
  A. increased pulmonary vasculature
  B. normal lung parenchyma
  C. heart size may be normal on x-ray in the first 24 hours of life
  D. the presence of moderate to gross cardiomegaly developing in rapid sequence on x-ray
  E. absence of the left ventricle

567. As pulmonary vascular resistance falls in the neonate with ventricular septal defect, all of the following may be observed EXCEPT
  A. the magnitude of left-to-right shunt increases
  B. congestive failure may occur
  C. tachypnea and rales may develop
  D. cyanosis becomes apparent
  E. cardiomegaly may be apparent on x-ray

568. The feature of ventricular septal defect that is most important in determining symptomatology is the
  A. age of the patient
  B. location of the defect in the septum
  C. number of defects
  D. size of defect and amount of left-to-right shunt
  E. sex of the patient

569. The signs and symptoms of an infant with a ventricular septal defect of moderate size include all of the following EXCEPT
   A. tachypnea and dyspnea
   B. feeding difficulties
   C. slow growth
   D. higher risk for pulmonary infection
   E. intermittent cyanosis

570. The occurrence of subacute bacterial endocarditis (SBE) in ventricular septal defect is
   A. less than 1%
   B. 10%
   C. 30%
   D. 20%
   E. 50%

571. The percentage of small ventricular septal defects estimated to close is
   A. 20% to 30%
   B. 50% to 80%
   C. 90% to 95%
   D. less than 5%
   E. 10% to 20%

572. The patient with a ventricular septal defect is considered inoperable if
   A. heart failure occurs in first month of life
   B. pulmonary hypertension is present
   C. marked cyanosis is present
   D. multiple defects are present in septum
   E. transposition of great arteries accompanies defect

573. The most common clinical manifestation of ventricular septal defect is
   A. signs of congestive heart failure in the first week of life
   B. small septal defects with trivial left-to-right shunt
   C. cyanosis
   D. chronic bronchitis
   E. moderate left-to-right shunting at the atrial level

574. All of the following are important in the prevention of sub-acute bacterial endocarditis in patients with ventricular septal defect EXCEPT
   A. the condition of the teeth
   B. the use of antibiotics for dental extraction
   C. the use of antibiotics for tonsillectomy
   D. early use of antibiotics for bacterial infections of the respiratory tract
   E. monthly injections of long-acting penicillin

575. In what percent of normal hearts does permanent anatomic closure of the foramen ovale occur?
   A. 95%
   B. 80%
   C. 70%
   D. 100%
   E. 50%

576. Some degree of cyanosis may be present in patients with patent foramen ovale in all of the following situations EXCEPT
   A. when pulmonary stenosis coexists
   B. when the patient has pulmonary hypertension
   C. when the right atrial pressure is increased
   D. when the tricuspid valve is stenotic
   E. when a ventricular septal defect is present

DIRECTIONS: For each of the questions or incomplete statements below, **ONE** or **MORE** of the answers or completions given is correct. Select
   A if only *1, 2 and 3* are correct,
   B if only *1 and 3* are correct,
   C if only *2 and 4* are correct,
   D if only *4* is correct,
   E if all are correct.

---

577. A list of structures derived from the endocardial cushion would include
   1. lowermost portion of the atrial septum
   2. portions of the septal leaflet of the mitral valve
   3. portions of the septal leaflet of the tricuspid valve
   4. lowermost portion of the ventricular septum

578. Changes in cardiac output and distribution of blood flow shortly after birth include
    1. rapid rise in cardiac output per kg body weight over the first three months
    2. sharp fall in pulmonary blood flow
    3. rapid rise in right ventricular output
    4. rapid fall in pulmonary arterial pressure

579. Factors that are thought to contribute to maintaining the patency of the ductus arteriosus are
    1. increased pulmonary vascular resistance secondary to hypoxia
    2. high arterial oxygen tension
    3. prostaglandin
    4. acetylcholine

580. The echocardiograph can be used to
    1. diagnose myocardial infarction
    2. determine the presence of a pericardial effusion
    3. distinguish a pathologic from an innocent murmur
    4. demonstrate the relationships of the great vessels to other cardiac structures

581. In second degree AV block
    1. every atrial impulse is conducted to the ventricle
    2. the outcome is usually fatal
    3. tachycardia frequently occurs
    4. there is almost always underlying heart disease

582. Cardiac lesions that can cause left-to-right shunts include
    1. patent ductus arteriosus
    2. anomalous origin of left coronary artery
    3. ventricular septal defect
    4. sinus of Valsalva fistula

583. In ventricular septal defect
    1. the murmur is generally harsh and of plateau type
    2. the smaller the defect, the greater the likelihood of spontaneous closure
    3. a mid-diastolic rumble may occur
    4. right-to-left shunting of blood is not a part of the natural course of the disease

Directions Summarized				
A	B	C	D	E
1,2,3	1,3	2,4	4	All are
only	only	only	only	correct

584. Tetralogy of Fallot includes
   1. right ventricular hypertrophy
   2. pulmonary outflow tract obstruction
   3. ventricular septal defect
   4. aortic stenosis

585. Metabolic derrangements that may affect myocardial function include
   1. Pompe's disease
   2. Hunter's syndrome
   3. hemachromatosis
   4. cystinosis

586. Acute pericarditis is manifested by
   1. pain
   2. a friction rub
   3. electrocardiographic changes
   4. arrhythmias

XII: Circulatory System
Answers and Comments

540. D. There is a functional closure of the foramen ovale at birth and an anatomic closure at approximately four months of age. *(REF. 1 — p. 1409)*

541. E. Bronchopneumonia would not be detectable by this technique, since it usually does not cause significant lung volume changes. *(REF. 2 — p. 1249)*

542. C. The first heart sound is increased in high cardiac output states. This sound is related to events occurring in early systole, and factors other than closure of the atrioventricular valves contribute. These include the rapid rise in isometric contraction. *(REF. 2 — p. 1249)*

543. D. The Valsalva maneuver usually causes the innocent murmur to disappear. *(REF. 3 — p. 1002)*

544. D. The venous hum will change with positioning changes of head or light compression over veins in neck. *(REF. 2 — p. 1251)*

545. E. A pulse rate of 260 in the presence of vigorous crying is considered cause for further investigation and observation. *(REF. 2 — p. 1252)*

546. D. Blood pressure is normally higher in the legs; flush pressure is an index of mean arterial pressure; and blood pressure varies considerably with age. A cuff that is too large for the extremity will produce falsely low readings. *(REF. 2 — pp. 1252–1253)*

547. C. The transverse diameter of the heart is approximately 7% to 8% of body height. *(REF. 2 — p. 1254)*

548. E. Newborn's at rest have a relatively high oxygen consumpton, which is associated with their relatively high cardiac output. *(REF. 2 — p. 1270)*

549. B. Oxygen saturation is almost 85% in fetal circulation. *(REF. 3 — p. 1018)*

550. A. The incidence of cardiovascular malformation at birth is approximately eight per 1,000. *(REF. 2 — p. 1272)*

551. B. Fifty percent of deaths related to congenital defects in the first year of life are cardiac in origin. *(REF. 2 — p. 1272)*

552. C. Patent ductus arteriosus and pulmonary arterial branch stenosis are associated with congenital rubella. *(REF. 2 — p. 1272)*

553. E. All of these factors except maternal psychotic illness have been associated with an increased risk of congenital heart disease in the neonate. *(REF. 2 — pp. 1272–1273)*

554. E. Generally only one of a pair of twins is affected by congenital heart disease. *(REF. 2 — p. 1273)*

555. D. Klinefelter's syndrome is not known to be associated with an increased incidence of congenital heart disease to the extent that the other syndromes are. *(REF. 2 — p. 1274)*

556. E. Pulmonary stenosis is the lesion exhibited by the patient with tetralogy of Fallot. *(REF. 2 — p. 1275)*

557. C. Cyanosis may not be present at birth and is best explained by patency of the ductus arteriosus. *(REF. 2 — p. 1275)*

558. A. Attacks may be spontaneous and unpredictable. *(REF. 2 — pp. 1275–1276)*

559. C. Bacterial endocarditis is rare in unoperated patients but is common in children who have had a palliative shunt procedure during infancy. *(REF. 2 — p. 1278)*

560. C. Of all the cyanotic lesions encountered in the first year of life, transposition of the great arteries has the highest mortality. Ventricular septal defects occur in about 50% of patients. Males are predominantly affected. Marked increases of pulmonary vascular resistance is generally found in older children. Polycythemia associated with transposition of the great vessels is usual in older infants. *(REF. 2 — pp. 1284–1285)*

561. E. Repair of ventricular defects is contraindicated as part of an emergency surgical approach since this might reduce blood mixture further. *(REF. 2 — pp. 1286–1287)*

562. E. Significant cardiomegaly is unusual in the neonate with isolated transposition of the great arteries. *(REF. 2 — p. 1286)*

563. C. The patient with a large VSD and transposition carries a poor prognosis. Cyanosis may be subtle and frequently delayed in onset. *(REF. 2 — p. 1288)*

564. D. The right atrium is enormous, and the size of the right ventricle is reduced in patients with Ebstein's disease. *(REF. 2 — pp. 1289–1290)*

565. D. All peripheral pulses are weak or impalpable in hypoplastic left heart syndrome. *(REF. 2 — p. 1292)*

566. E. Evaluation of left ventricular size is difficult on plain x-ray because of the cardiomegaly that progresses rapidly. *(REF. 2 — p. 1292)*

567. D. Cyanosis is not a feature at this point in the course of the disease. *(REF. 2 — pp. 1295–1296)*

568. D. Blood flow through the defect is the major determinant of cardiac dysfunction *(REF. 2 — p. 1292)*

569. E. All but intermittent cyanosis may occur, and the infants may suffer recurrent pulmonary infections with or without congestive cardiac failure. *(REF. 2 — p. 1296)*

570. A. Less than 1% developed SBE as a complication. *(REF. 2 — p. 1297)*

571. B. Most of these do so by the first year of life, but closure may occur even in later years. *(REF. 2 — p. 1297)*

572. C. Infants with large right-to-left shunt causing marked cyanosis are considered inoperable. *(REF. 2 — p. 1298)*

573. B. Most patients with VSD have small defects and are asymptomatic. *(REF. 2 — p. 1296)*

574. E. Prophylactic, long-acting penicillin therapy is not warranted, since the incidence of SBE is low in these patients. *(REF. 2 — p. 1297)*

575. B. In about 20% of normal hearts a small slit-like opening will persist. *(REF. 2 — p. 1300)*

576. E. Without increased right atrial pressure no shunt will occur, and the presence of a smaller moderate-sized VSD would not be expected to produce cyanosis. *(REF. 2 — p. 1300)*

577. A. The endocardial cushion makes up the lowermost portion of the atrial septum, the uppermost portion of the ventricular septum, and portions of the septal leaflets of the tricuspid and mitral valves. *(REF. 1 — p. 1356)*

578. D. Shortly after birth there is an initial rise in CO but over the next three months the CO falls slowly. The RV output remains approximately the same. Pulmonary arterial blood flow rises sharply, and pulmonary arterial pressure falls. *(REF. 1 — p. 1354)*

579. B. The ductus arteriosus is kept open by prostaglandins and by hypoxia-induced pulmonary hypertension. The ductus is closed by high arterial oxygen tensions and acetylcholine. *(REF. 1 — p. 1354)*

580. C. The echocardiograph can be used to detect the presence of pericardial fluid and to demonstrate the relationships of the great vessels to each other and other structures. The echocardiogram cannot diagnose MI nor can it distinguish murmurs. *(REF. 1 — p. 1369)*

581. D. In second degree AV block there is almost always underlying acute or chronic heart disease, and therefore it deserves thorough investigation. The ventricular rate is usually slow, and the block is at the level of the AV node and His system, thus sometimes blocking beats generated in the atria from reaching the ventricle. The condition is not usually fatal, since the advent of treatment with pacemakers. *(REF. 1 — p. 1402)*

582. E. All of cardiac lesions listed have the creation of a left-to-right shunting of blood as a pathological feature. *(REF. 1 — p. 1404)*

583. A. In VSD, the murmur is of a harsh quality and of the plateau type, but if the ratio of pulmonary to systemic flow is 2:1 then a diastolic rumble can occur. Many of the smaller VSDs close spontaneously. If the shunt is significant and unrelieved by surgery, then pulmonary hypertension can occur with a resulting right-to-left shunting of blood. *(REF. 1 — p. 1414)*

584. A. Tetralogy of Fallot is made up of an overriding aorta, VSD, RVH, and pulmonary outflow tract obstruction. Aortic stenosis is not a feature of this syndrome. *(REF. 1 — p. 1447)*

585. E. The myocardium is damaged by glycogen in Pompe's disease, by hemosiderin deposition in hemochromatosis, by cystine crystals in cystinosis, and by degeneration in the mucopolysaccharidosis (Hunter's and Hurler's syndrome). *(REF. 1 — p. 1473)*

586. A. Acute pericarditis is manifested by pain, S-T segment elevation on ECG, a friction rub, and sometimes fever. Arrhythmias can occur in pancarditis but are not a feature of acute pericarditis alone. *(REF. 1 — p. 1474)*

XIII: Nervous System

587. Chorea is more often associated with
    A. idiosyncracy to phenothiazines
    B. forms of encephalitis
    C. hepatolenticular degeneration
    D. dystonia musculorum
    E. rheumatic fever

588. An infant born at 34 weeks gestation would be LEAST likely to exhibit the
    A. Moro reflex
    B. grasp reflex
    C. suck reflex
    D. automatic walk
    E. pupillary response

589. All of the following are characteristic of agenesis of the corpus callosum EXCEPT
    A. it usually presents as a triad of symptoms: nystagmus, flattened nasal bridge, and dull affect
    B. with simple nondecussation of the corpus callosum fibers, the patient leads a normal life
    C. it may be associated with heteropias, holoprosencephaly, or destructive lesions
    D. corpus callosum is a large bundle of nerve fibers connecting cortex of one cerebral hemisphere with the other
    E. there is no specific test other than x-ray contrast studies

590. Probably the most frequent cause of hydrocephalus is
    A. spina bifida with meningomyelocele
    B. postinflammatory or posttraumatic obstruction
    C. Dandy-Walker syndrome
    D. neoplasm (glioma in the third ventricle)
    E. Arnold-Chiari malformation

591. All of the following are true statements regarding anencephaly EXCEPT
    A. it is the most common CNS malformation incompatible with life
    B. it is six times more common in whites than blacks
    C. it is three times more common in males than females
    D. the mother often has hydramnios
    E. the diagnosis can be made prepartum by x-ray of the abdomen

592. Medical treatment for Down's syndrome includes
    A. special diets low in carotene and food additives
    B. thyroid extract
    C. megavitamins
    D. 5-hydroxytryptophan
    E. no specific medical therapy

593. Spastic cerebral palsy (spastic hemiplegia) is associated with all of the following EXCEPT
    A. the patient characteristically walks on heels
    B. there is increased tone with tightness of adductors of the thigh
    C. there are signs of upper motor neuron involvement
    D. the involved extremities may be shorter in length
    E. the involved hand may show astereognosis

594. Which of the following is most frequently associated with cerebral palsy?
    A. Blindness
    B. Seizure disorders
    C. Deafness and hypacusis
    D. Hydrocephalus
    E. Horner's syndrome

595. Which of the following is NOT true of increased intracranial pressure associated with a brain tumor?
    A. Headache site is of value in localizing tumor
    B. Cranial enlargement can result from obstructive hydrocephalus
    C. Vomiting tends to occur on arising
    D. Double vision can result from sixth nerve palsy
    E. Papilledema may not be present

596. All of the following are associated with cerebellar astrocytoma EXCEPT
    A. no age group is exempt, but peak incidence is from 5 to 8 years of age
    B. the majority of patients are symptomatic less than two months prior to diagnosis
    C. there are signs and symptoms of increased intracranial pressure
    D. ataxia predominates on one side
    E. nystagmus and head tilt are present

597. Medulloblastoma is usually NOT associated with
    A. signs and symptoms similar to cerebellar astrocytoma
    B. onset usually more acute than with cerebellar astrocytoma
    C. seizures
    D. rapid course
    E. poor prognosis

598. Regarding tumors of the optic nerve and chiasm all of the following are true EXCEPT
    A. almost all of these tumors are gliomas
    B. diminished visual acuity is common
    C. exophthalmos is rare
    D. there is proptosis of a mild degree
    E. there is optic atrophy

599. Which of the following is NOT characteristic of craniopharyngioma?
    A. Evidences of increased intracranial pressure
    B. Presence of visual defects
    C. Endocrine dysfunctions, diminished pituitary activity
    D. Growth retardation
    E. Diabetes insipidus in over 50% of cases

600. The most frequent symptoms of intraspinal tumors in children is (are)
A. disturbances of gait and posture
B. pain
C. decreased deep tendon reflexes
D. enuresis and encopresis
E. a bruit over the vertebral column

601. Pseudotumor cerebri is characterized by all of the following, EXCEPT
A. increased intracranial pressure
B. convulsions and impaired mentation
C. blurred vision and diplopia
D. florid papilledema and abducens nerve paresis
E. no consistent signs of neurologic dysfunction

602. A seven-year-old child presents with seizures, depressed sensorium, focal motor deficits, and signs of circulatory stasis. Temperature is elevated. An abscess of the nose is found. The most likely diagnosis is
A. fat embolism
B. periarteritis nodosa
C. venous thromboses
D. dissecting cerebral aneurysm
E. pseudotumor cerebri

603. The most lethal complication of head injury is
A. extradural hemorrhage
B. meningitis
C. subdural hematoma
D. convulsive disorder
E. concussion

604. Regarding extradural hematoma all of the following are true EXCEPT
A. it is most common in children less than two years of age
B. it is the most lethal complication of head injury; untreated mortality about 100%
C. there is no mechanism for absorption of an extradural hemorrhage, and, therefore, there is a rapid rise in intracranial pressure
D. treatment is surgical
E. untreated cases survive only two to three days

605. All of the following are usually associated with closed head injuries in children EXCEPT
   A. transient loss of consciousness may follow sudden head blow
   B. convulsions mean severe brain damage
   C. transient loss of vision may occur
   D. children may vomit after injury
   E. they may be managed at home if parents can check size of pupils, motor strength, and responsiveness

606. A 14 - and six-per-second positive spike dysrhythmia during light sleep, on EEG, suggests
   A. grand mal seizure
   B. absence seizure (petit mal)
   C. hypsarhythmia or massive myoclonic seizure
   D. psychomotor epilepsy
   E. none of the above

607. Petit mal (absence attacks) are usually characterized by all of the following EXCEPT
   A. attacks rarely last more than five to 15 seconds
   B. typically the child abruptly recovers senses
   C. there is usually no aura
   D. frequency may be increased by fatigue, photic stimulation, and emotional stress
   E. EEG is not characteristic

608. Clinical manifestations of acute polyneuritis include all of the following EXCEPT
   A. mild to profound paresis, usually ascending and symmetrical
   B. bilateral facial nerve paresis
   C. paresthesias are common
   D. partial or complete absence of deep tendon reflexes
   E. increased CSF pressure, elevated cell count to 3,000 monocytes

609. All of the following are characteristic of subacute sclerosing panencephalitis (SSPE) EXCEPT
   A. it is a disease of children and young adults
   B. seizures are a late manifestation and are of the absence type
   C. gamma globulin is increased in CSF
   D. there is a strong association of SSPE with measles virus
   E. it predominantly affects boys

610. All of the following are characteristic of psychomotor seizures EXCEPT
   A. they are most difficult to recognize and control
   B. purposeful, repetitive, inappropriate motor acts
   C. fugue states and episodes of confusion are rare
   D. they are usually not associated with tonic or clonic movements
   E. the EEG is abnormal at all times, revealing temporal lobe slow waves and spikes between seizures

611. Infantile myoclonic seizures
   A. have also been called petit mal seizures
   B. usually involve a single muscle group
   C. may recur several hundred times a day
   D. are very difficult to differentiate from pyknolepsy on EEG
   E. are best treated with phenobarbital

612. Infants with grand mal seizures are best treated with
   A. phenobarbital
   B. mephobarbital
   C. phenytoin
   D. trimethadione
   E. ethosuximide

613. As part of the neurologic examination of a five-year-old child, behavior and mental status are assessed. Which of the following appears to be an abnormal finding?
   A. Can follow three part commands
   B. Can draw a figure with more than five recognizable parts
   C. Has not developed preference for one hand in writing and eating
   D. Can speak fluently
   E. May not have learned to identify colors

614. All of the following relate to disorders of movement EXCEPT
  A. chorea associated with diseases of the basal ganglia
  B. athetosis associated with diseases of the basal ganglia
  C. dystonia associated with diseases of the basal ganglia
  D. intention tremor associated with diseases of the basal ganglia
  E. tremors associated with thyrotoxicosis

615. A child presents with bitemporal hemianopsia. The most likely diagnosis is a lesion in
  A. the optic radiation of the visual cortex
  B. the region of the optic chiasm
  C. the optic tract
  D. the optic nerve
  E. the temporal lobe

616. A 14-month-old has a lumbar puncture performed for suspected meningitis. All of the following values are normal findings EXCEPT
  A. faint xanthochromia
  B. no red blood cells
  C. protein of 15 mg/dl
  D. spinal fluid glucose was half that of blood glucose
  E. two leukocytes

617. Spina bifida with meningomyelocele
  A. usually occurs in the thoracic region
  B. is a rare anomaly of the nervous system
  C. is best treated with conservative medical management until age six months
  D. may not be apparent until the child is ready to walk
  E. is none of the above

618. All of the following are true of spasmus nutans EXCEPT
  A. it is usually first noticed between ages four and 12 months
  B. there are intermittent rapid pendular nystagmoid movements with head nodding
  C. it is caused by maldevelopment and small size of the occipital lobe
  D. it must be distinguished from searching nystagmus
  E. surgery is not indicated

619. "Migraine" in children is characterized by
  A. absence of an aura
  B. onset in early childhood
  C. negative family history
  D. unrelated to stress
  E. relief of attack by sleep

620. A 12-year-old girl presents with a chief complaint of ptosis and double vision. Examination reveals weakness of the extraocular, neck, and facial muscles. Progressive weakness is noted on repetitive or sustained muscular contractions. When the patient maintains an upward gaze, a progressive ptosis is noted. Muscle weakness improves with rest. Thyroid studies are normal. The most likely diagnosis is
  A. Bell palsy
  B. juvenile myasthenia gravis
  C. congenital ptosis
  D. congenital facial nerve palsy
  E. myositis ossificans progressiva

621. Congenital muscular dystrophy
  A. is caused by a sex-linked gene
  B. occurs at ages 12 to 18 months
  C. is associated with hyperreflexia
  D. is associated with fasciculations of the tongue
  E. is associated with none of the above

DIRECTIONS: This sections consists of situations, each followed by a series of questions. Study each situation, and select the **one** best answer to each question following it.

CASE 1 (Questions 622-623): A four and one-half year-old boy has a four-month history of increasing neurologic disorders. The findings include paresis of conjugate gaze, hemiparesis and hyperreflexia, Babinski response, horizontal nystagmus, and truncal and extremity ataxia. The child does NOT exhibit sensory deficits. Basal ganglia manifestations are NOT detected. CSF pressure, cell count, protein, and sugar are normal. Plain x-rays of the skull are normal.

622. At this point the diagnosis is probably
A. Sydenham's chorea
B. meningitis
C. pinealoma
D. agenesis of the corpus callosum
E. none of the above

623. Pneumoencephalogram and computerized axial tomography reveal a posterior and upward displacement of the aqueduct of Sylvius and the fourth ventricle. Now the most likely diagnosis is a
A. brainstem glioma
B. pinealoma
C. thalamic tumor
D. ependymoma
E. astrocytoma

CASE 2 (Questions 624-625): A 15-year-old boy is in a motorcycle accident in which he is struck by a car. The child sustains a closed head injury and minor orthopedic injuries. The patient remains unconscious for three days followed by several days of stupor. During the three days of coma, the child exhibited difficulty with respiration and a convulsion. Cerebral edema is strongly suspected.

624. Which of the following would be of LEAST value in management of the patient during the three days of coma?
A. CSF studies
B. IV fluids and electrolyte studies
C. Endotracheal intubation
D. Treatment with phenytoin
E. Dexamethasone therapy

The patient is discharged from the hospital after 15 days without medications. However, the parents are concerned about seizures developing later as a result of the injury.

625. All of the following are correct in counseling EXCEPT

    A. late epilepsy occurs in less than 5% of cases of closed head injuries

    B. seizures may occur; peak incidence occurs at six to 18 months after injury

    C. the EEG can be used to accurately predict the chances of epilepsy after the injury

    D. some patients are maintained on medications for at least two years, but no absolute criteria have been established

    E. penetrating depressed fractures have a seizure incidence of 30% to 60% when associated with prolonged unconsciousness

CASE 3 (Questions 626-627): A three-year-old had myoclonic seizures during infancy and later developed grand mal and psychomotor seizures. He was presumed to be mentally retarded, was hyperactive, and destructive and displayed bright red and brown nodules in a butterfly distribution over nose and cheeks. The child died, and autopsy revealed sclerotic patches scattered throughout the gray matter of the cerebral cortex. These patches consisted of astrocytes and bizarre giant cells. Calcium was found in some of the patches. Small tumors made up of fibrous tissue, fat, smooth muscle, and blood vessels were found in the kidney, heart, and liver.

626. The most likely diagnosis in this case is

    A. tuberous sclerosis

    B. malignant glioblastoma

    C. miliary tuberculosis

    D. chronic lymphocytic leukemia

    E. lupus erythematosus

627. Although not described, examination of the eye would probably have revealed

    A. ptosis of the eyelids

    B. cataracts

    C. coarse nystagmus

    D. visual acuity of 20/200

    E. retinal lesions

DIRECTIONS: Each set of lettered headings below is followed by a list of numbered words or phrases. For each numbered word or phrase select

        A if the item is associated with (A) *only*,
        B if the item is associated with (B) *only*,
        C if the item is associated with *both* (A) *and* (B),
        D if the item is associated with *neither* (A) *nor* (B).

    A. Cerebellar astrocytoma
    B. Medulloblastoma
    C. Both
    D. Neither

628. The most common posterior fossa tumor in children

629. Treatment and diagnosis involve surgery

630. Long-term survival is characteristically poor

631. Radiotherapy is not helpful

632. May present with signs of increased intracranial pressure

    A. Subdural hematoma
    B. Extradural hematomas
    C. Both
    D. Neither

633. May exist without skull fractures

634. High incidence in children less than one year of age

635. Subhyaloid hemorrhages occur

636. May occur from venous bleeding

637. The most lethal complication of head injury

    A. Myasthenia gravis
    B. Congenital myotonia
    C. Both
    D. Neither

638. Seldom involves muscles of respiration or swallowing

639. Neostigmine used in treatment

640. Muscular hypertrophy prominent

641. Variable mode of inheritance

642. Uniformly fatal in childhood

    A. Neurofibromatosis
    B. Sturge-Weber syndrome
    C. Both
    D. Neither

643. Autosomal dominant inheritance

644. High incidence of mental retardation

645. Ceroid lipofuscinosis is a common complication

646. Intracranial calcifications are pathognomonic

647. Manifestations of the disease involve the skin

    A. Lesch-Nyhan syndrome
    B. Huntington's chorea
    C. Both
    D. Neither

648. Involves a disorder of movement

649. Sex-linked recessive mode of inheritance

650. Manifests symptoms in most cases after childhood

651. Pathogenesis is unknown

652. Renal failure is common

XIII: Nervous System
Answers and Comments

587. E. Conditions A, B, C, and D are usually associated with involuntary sustained spasms of the muscles involving the neck, trunk, and extremities. These spasms may cause abnormal posturing. On the other hand, chorea, which is characterized by sudden, irregular jerking movements is associated with rheumatic fever (Sydenham's chorea) and can involve any skeletal muscle group including the face. *(REF. 1 — p. 1735)*

588. D. Automatic walk is absent in an infant at 32 weeks and minimal at 34 weeks. At 37 weeks this reflex is fair on toes; it is good on heels at 41 weeks. *(REF. 1 — p. 1738)*

589. A. There are no characteristic signs or symptoms. Most cases of agenesis of the corpus callosum present as accidental findings during a neurologic workup that utilizes contrast x-ray studies. *(REF. 1 — p. 1753)*

590. B. Postinflammatory or posttraumatic obstruction of the basilar cistern and subarachnoid pathways are the most common causes of hydrocephalus. Fibrosis secondary to intracranial bleeding at birth and meningitis can result in obstruction. *(REF. 1 — p. 1754)*

591. C. The frequency of occurrence in female fetuses and prematures may be as high as seven times that encountered in males. *(REF. 1 — p. 1757)*

592. E. There is no specific medical treatment for this disorder. Therapy is supportive including educational, vocational and social planning. Drug therapy has been of little value in improving intellect or muscle tone. *(REF. 1 — p. 1778)*

593. A. Characteristically the patient with spastic hemiplegia will walk more on the toes than the heels. This results in a circumduction of the affected leg in order to compensate for the apparent lengthening. *(REF. 1 — pp. 1780, 1781)*

594. B. The most commonly associated problems are convulsions and mental retardation. Convulsions occur in approximately 25% to 35% of all children with cerebral palsy. Seizures appear to be more common in postnatally acquired cerebral palsy. *(REF. 1 — p. 1782)*

595. A. Headache in children may not be a reliable nor a localizing sign for brain tumor. Headache may be intermittent. Frequency of headache is unrelated to site, i.e., supratentorial or infratentorial. *(REF. 1 — p. 1804)*

596. B. Cerebellar astrocytoma in childhood has a relatively "quiet" onset and is slowly progressive. The majority of children have symptoms two to seven months before diagnosis. In some children this latent period may be several years. *(REF. 1 — p. 1807)*

597. C. Seizures are not common with medulloblastoma. When they do occur they probably represent seeding of the tumor on the cerebral hemispheres. *(REF. 1 — p. 1808)*

598. C. Exophthalmos is an early and a frequent sign when the tumor is confirned to one optic nerve. *(REF. 1 — p. 1814)*

599. E. Diabetes insipidus is an uncommon complication of craniopharyngioma. Other manifestations of hypothalamic dysfunction are more common: growth retardation, obesity, etc. These usually appear postoperatively; somatic and sexual infantilism occur preoperatively. *(REF. 1 — p. 1816)*

600. A. The changes in gait and posture are caused by weakness, spasticity, and/or an attempt to avoid pain. There is a tendency to avoid flexing the trunk. Paraspinal muscle spasm occurs; gait disturbances reflect lower extremity involvement and changes in muscle tone. *(REF. 1 — pp. 1817, 1818)*

601. B. Pseudotumor cerebri is a syndrome caused by intracranial hypertension (etiology and pathogenesis are not fully understood). Convulsions and alterations of the mental state do not occur and suggest that the underlying mechanism is unrelated to cerebral edema. *(REF. 1 — pp. 1819, 1820)*

602. C. Venous occlusion may be associated with the abscess of the nose. The clinical picture depends on the rapidity and extent of the occlusion. The signs and symptoms presented are compatible with venous thromboses. *(REF. 1 — pp. 1821, 1822)*

603. A. Untreated extradural hemorrhage has a 100% mortality; it is almost 50% in surgically treated patients. When untreated, death may occur in two to three days. *(REF. 1 — p. 1830)*

604. A. Extradural hemorrhage (hematoma) is not common in children less than two years of age because, anatomically, the vessels are less adherent to the skull. The hematoma is a result of bleeding between dura mater and skull. It is often associated with a tear in the middle meningeal artery. *(REF. 1 — p. 1830)*

605. B. Convulsions may occur with closed head injuries and do *not* necessarily imply severe brain pathology. Convulsions may occur as a result of profuse cerebral stimuli. A seizure at the time of injury does not prognosticate future convulsions. *(REF. 1 — p. 1831)*

606. E. This EEG pattern is believed to arise in the diencephalic nuclei and/or limbic system. The meaning is still controversial. Some believe it represents a "seizure equivalent." However, the finding has been detected in a large percentage of clinically normal children. The true pathologic significance is unknown. *(REF. 1 — p. 1839)*

607. E. The EEG in petit mal is very characteristic, usually revealing bursts of generalized bilaterally synchronous three-per-second spike and wave complexes. These occur against a background of relatively normal activity. *(REF. 1 — p. 1844)*

608. E. The CSF findings are characteristic: pressure is usually normal, cell count is usually normal, sugar is normal and protein elevated. The observation of elevated protein and normal cell count was described by Guillain, Barré and Strohl. *(REF. 1 — pp. 1865, 1866)*

609. B. Myoclonic seizures are an early manifestation of SSPE. Affected children lapse into sustained and continuous seizures and may become comatose, spastic, and decorticate. *(REF. 1 — p. 1880)*

610. E. The EEG may be normal except at the time of the psychomotor seizure. *(REF. 2 — p. 1719)*

611. C. Only choice C is correct. Infantile myoclonic seizures have also been called "infantile spasms" or "jacknife epilepsy." They occur usually before two years of age and involve more than a single group of muscles. The EEG changes are characteristic, revealing random high-voltage slow waves and spikes. The pattern has been termed hypsarhythmia. The drug of choice is a corticosteroid or pyridoxine. *(REF. 2 — p. 1719)*

612. A. Phenobarbital is the drug of choice for most patients with grand mal epilepsy. Phenytoin cannot be administered in suspension form to infants because small doses are difficult to administer accurately; it is, however, a good choice to control grand mal seizures. Trimethadione is best used in the treatment of petit mal epilepsy or absence attacks. Ethosuximide is also used for absence attacks. *(REF. 2 — pp. 1724-1725)*

613. C. Preference for one hand or the other is usually established by age three years. Cerebral dominance for left or right-hand preference may be delayed in children with mental retardation or learning disabilities. *(REF. 2 — pp. 1731-1732)*

614. D. All of the conditions as cited are correct regarding abnormal motor movements except for D. Tremors may be seen with a variety of disorders: anxiety, thyrotoxicosis, Wilson's disease. Intention tremor is a sign of cerebellar involvement and is not caused by disease of the basal ganglia. The disorders of the extrapyramidal system disappear during sleep. *(REF. 2 — pp. 1733-1734)*

615. B. Bitemporal hemianopsia implies a lesion interrupting fibers to the nasal half of both retina. The anatomic position would be at the optic chiasm, and is seen most often in children with a craniopharyngioma. A lesion in the optic tract causes homonymous hemianopsia. A lesion in the optic nerve causes unilateral visual loss. *(REF. 2 — p. 1735)*

616. A. Xanthochromia is abnormal under any condition in a 14-month-old. It may represent elevated spinal fluid protein, bilirubin accumulation, or it may be a result of bleeding. *(REF. 2 — pp. 1741-1742)*

617. E. Spina bifida with meningomyelocele is one of the more common neurologic developmental anomalies. It represents a midline defect of skull, vertebral arches, and neural tube. Evident at birth, usually over the lumbosacral region, the defect is usually covered by membrane with neural tissue attached. Most defects are associated with Arnold-Chiari malformations. Surgical closure is recommended within 48 hours to prevent infection and meningitis. *(REF. 2 — pp. 1748-1749)*

618. C. The etiology of spasmus nutans is unknown. Examination reveals no pathognomonic pathology. Therapy is not indicated; spontaneous improvement is the rule. *(REF. 2 — p. 1758)*

619. E. Migraine is believed to be a common cause of vascular headache in children. A positive family history is found in about two thirds of patients. The onset is usually in the older child or adolescent. The characteristic aura may include visual disturbances or other transitory neurologic disturbances. Stress increases the number of attacks; sleep relieves the attack. *(REF. 2 — p. 1762)*

620. B. The diagnosis is based on the observation of progressive weakness on sustained muscular contraction. The progressive ptosis on sustained upward gaze is a good example of this. The sex and age also support the diagnosis. Myositis ossificans progressiva occurs primarily in males. The initial feature may be a torticollis with onset occurring from birth to late childhood. It is usually associated with congenital malformations. The facial nerve palsy is associated with selective weakness of muscles innervated by the mandibular branch, causing paralysis of the lower lip and angle of the mouth. Bell palsy is associated with facial weakness and pain in the ear on the affected side. The face is pulled toward the normal side. Congenital ptosis causes drooping of one or both eyelids, which is noted during the neonatal period. It is not associated with double vision or the other symptoms reported. *(REF. 2 — p. 1802)*

621. E. Congenital muscular dystrophy is an autosomal recessive disorder. The onset occurs in utero and as a result muscle atrophy and contractures are present at birth. Unlike Werdnig-Hoffmann disease, tongue fasciculations do not occur. The deep tendon reflexes are depressed. *(REF. 2 — p. 1808)*

622. E. The signs and symptoms described are characteristic of none of the items listed. The neurologic findings are most suggestive of brainstem pathology. There is evidence of pyramidal tract and cerebellar pathway involvement, as well as cranial nerve involvement. *(REF. 1 — p. 1810)*

623. A. The air study and CAT scan in combination with the clinical findings are almost diagnostic of the brainstem glioma. This tumor constitutes 10% of all intracranial tumors in children. *(REF. 1 — p. 1810)*

624. A. The CSF studies will probably be of little value. The study during the initial acute traumatic period will not be helpful in differentiating extradural, subdural, or intracortical bleeding. Elevated CSF pressure is anticipated. Findings would not determine the course of therapy. *(REF. 1 — pp. 1832, 1833)*

625. C. The EEG is not too reliable a prognostic indicator. Gross irregularity of the EEG after head trauma can be found in a normal child. A normal EEG three months after injury tends to make post-traumatic epilepsy less likely. A worsening EEG makes one suspicious. The EEG may be a misleading laboratory method of predicting epilepsy posttrauma. *(REF. 1 — p. 1833)*

626. A. The diagnosis of tuberous sclerosis is strongly suggested by the combined clinical signs. The seizures, retardation, destructive behaviors, and aggressiveness are common as is the changing pattern of seizures characteristic. Skin lesions (adenoma sebaceum) are found in 80% of patients. Confirmation is made by the description of the pathologic lesions. *(REF. 2 — pp. 1763–1764)*

627. E. The characteristic lesions in about half of the patients are retinal. They appear as elevated yellow or white areas usually near the edge of the optic disc. The lesions are malformations of the nerve fiber layer of the retina. and as a rule do not impair visual acuity. *(REF. 2 — pp. 1763–1764)*

628. B. Both medulloblastoma and cerebellar astrocytoma may
629. C. present with signs of increased intracranial pressure.
630. B. Medulloblastoma is the most common posterior fossa
631. D. tumor and carries a poor long-term prognosis. The treat-
632. C. ment and diagnosis of both tumors involves surgery, and
both respond favorably to radiotherapy. *(REF. 1 — p. 1808)*

633. C. Both subdural hematoma and extradural hematoma may
634. A. exist without skull fracture and both can occur from
635. C. venous bleeds. Subhyaloid hemorrhages occur in both con-
636. C. ditions also. Subdural hematoma is more common in chil-
637. B. dren less than one year of age. Extradural hematomas are
the most lethal complication of head injury. *(REF. 1 — p. 1830)*

638. B. Congenital myotonia is inherited by a variable mode and
639. A. seldom affects the muscles of respiration or swallowing;
640. B. muscular hypertrophy is prominent in this disorder.

641. B. Neostigmine is used in the treatment of myasthenia.
642. D. Neither condition is uniformly fatal in childhood. *(REF.
1 — pp. 1888, 1889)*

643. A. Both neurofibromatosis and the Sturge-Weber syndrome
644. B. have skin findings (café au lait spots and vascular nevi).
645. D. There is a high incidence of mental retardation in the
646. B. Sturge-Weber syndrome, and the intracranial calcifica-
647. C. tions are pathognomonic. Neither syndrome is associated
with ceroid lipofuscinosis. *(REF. 1 — p. 1930)*

648. C. Lesch-Nyhan syndrome is a sex-linked recessive abnor-
649. A. mality of purine metabolism in which there is a movement
650. B. disorder (chorea athetosis) and renal failure is common in
651. B. untreated subjects. Huntington's chorea is of unknown
652. A. pathogenesis and as the name implies, involves a movement disorder. The disease presents in 95% of patients
after the childhood years. *(REF. 1 — pp. 1925, 1926)*

XIV: Respiratory System

DIRECTIONS: Each of the questions or incomplete statements below is followed by five suggested answers or completions. Select the **one** that is **BEST** in each case.

---

653. Diabetes mellitus is more likely to develop in a patient with cystic fibrosis at age
    A. two years
    B. seven years
    C. 12 years
    D. 20 years
    E. one year

654. What percentage of patients with cystic fibrosis will be found to have liver cirrhosis at autopsy?
    A. 100%
    B. 50%
    C. 1%
    D. 75%
    E. 25%

655. The mode of inheritance of cystic fibrosis is
    A. autosomal recessive
    B. sex-linked recessive
    C. multifactorial
    D. undetermined
    E. autosomal dominant with variable penetrance

656. The increased appetite of patients with cystic fibrosis may be related to all of the following EXCEPT
  A. absence of pyloric reflex
  B. lack of free fatty acids in the duodenum
  C. failure of release of enterogastrone
  D. underdosage of pancreatic enzyme
  E. poor carbohydrate absorption

657. Patients with cystic fibrosis have sweat and chloride levels in the range of
  A. 5 to 50 mEq/L
  B. 200 to 300 mEq/L
  C. 40 to 70 mEq/L
  D. 5 to 10 mEq/L
  E. 70 to 180 mEq/L

658. What percentage of patients with cystic fibrosis have abnormal elevations of sodium and chloride in sweat?
  A. 77%
  B. 88%
  C. 50%
  D. 66%
  E. 99%

659. The cystic fibrosis patient with pancreatic insufficiency is usually most intolerant of
  A. fat
  B. protein
  C. monosaccharides
  D. starch
  E. disaccharides

660. The problem of fat malabsorption in cystic fibrosis can be treated by all of the following EXCEPT
  A. medium-chain triglycerides
  B. enzyme replacement
  C. reduction of the fat content of diet
  D. medium-chain triglycerides plus enzyme replacement
  E. long-chain triglyceride as fat source

661. The relative humidity of air after passage through the nasal passages is
    A. 40%
    B. 95%
    C. 70%
    D. 60%
    E. 80%

662. The most common congenital malformation of the nasal passages is
    A. choanal atresia
    B. benign polyps
    C. septal deviation
    D. dermoid tumor
    E. capillary hemangioma

663. The treatment for bilateral choanal atresia is
    A. puncture of obstruction at delivery
    B. establishment of oral airway
    C. intensive nasal mucosa vasoconstriction
    D. tracheostomy
    E. no treatment is necessary

664. Which of the following is the primary presenting complaint with foreign bodies in the nasal passages?
    A. Pain
    B. Bleeding from the nostril
    C. Watery discharge
    D. Ipsilateral "watery" eye
    E. Obstruction

665. The most common cause of nosebleed in children is
    A. trauma
    B. infection
    C. polyps
    D. allergic rhinitis
    E. nasal foreign body

666. A child who vomits blood each morning upon arising, but who has no other gastrointestinal complaints may have
  A. sinusitis
  B. adenoiditis
  C. nosebleeds
  D. peptic ulcer disease
  E. Meckel's diverticulum

667. Most acute respiratory tract infections in children are caused by
  A. streptococci
  B. viral agents
  C. viral agents and mycoplasma
  D. *H. influenzae*
  E. pneumococci

668. All of the following infectious agents may cause primary acute tonsillopharyngitis EXCEPT
  A. staphylococci
  B. streptococci
  C. viral agents
  D. diphtheria organisms
  E. *Neisseria gonorrhoeae*

669. The principal single cause of bronchiolitis is
  A. *H. influenzae*
  B. pneumococcus
  C. parainfluenza
  D. Coxsackie A
  E. respiratory syncytial virus

670. The principal single cause of croup syndrome is
  A. *H. influenzae*
  B. respiratory syncytial virus
  C. Coxsackie B
  D. parainfluenza virus
  E. group A streptococci

671. Respiratory tract disease in children is caused by influenza viruses which mainly occur
   A. during epidemics
   B. as sporadic cases
   C. in association with bacterial disease
   D. as croup syndrome
   E. in the spring months

672. In which of the following does mycoplasmal respiratory tract disease usually peak?
   A. Zero to one year
   B. Three to five years
   C. Five to seven years
   D. Late childhood and early adult life
   E. Neonatal age period

673. The principal agent responsible for the common cold is
   A. respiratory syncytial virus
   B. adenovirus
   C. Coxsackie virus
   D. parainfluenza virus
   E. rhinovirus

674. The frequency of colds in infancy appears to be most closely related to
   A. age
   B. allergic conditions in home
   C. number of exposures
   D. malnutrition
   E. presence or absence of anemia

675. The incidence of colds in normal children is
   A. one to two per year
   B. eight to ten per year
   C. six to eight per year
   D. ten to 15 per year
   E. three to six per year

676. The most common complication of acute nasopharyngitis in children is
   A. bronchitis
   B. sinusitis
   C. otitis media
   D. laryngitis
   E. pneumonia

677. The most distressing symptom of the common cold in children is
   A. fever
   B. myalgia
   C. headache
   D. ear pain
   E. nasal obstruction

678. In the majority of patients with colds, orally administered decongestants will
   A. reduce the incidence of otitis media
   B. prevent the spread of the process to the lower respiratory tract
   C. decrease the incidence of secondary bacterial infection
   D. cause sedation only
   E. do none of the above

679. In what percentage of nonepidemic cases of acute pharyngitis is group A beta-hemolytic streptococci the offending agent?
   A. 1%
   B. 10%
   C. 5%
   D. 2%
   E. 20%

680. The physical finding most likely to be associated with streptococcal pharyngitis is
   A. exudate on tonsils
   B. redness of tonsils
   C. lymphadenitis
   D. hoarseness
   E. "strawberry" tongue

681. The percentage of normal children who carry streptococci in their throats is
- **A.** 1% to 2%
- **B.** 5% to 10%
- **C.** 15% to 20%
- **D.** 20% to 25%
- **E.** 30% to 35%

682. Pharyngitis with conjunctivitis is most often caused by
- **A.** adenovirus
- **B.** Coxsackie virus
- **C.** *H. influenzae*
- **D.** group A strep
- **E.** *S. aureus*

683. The most common cause of retropharyngeal abscess is
- **A.** a penetrating injury of posterior pharyngeal wall
- **B.** dissection of purulent material from tonsil
- **C.** suppuration of draining nodes of retropharyngeal spaces
- **D.** tonsil and adenoid surgery
- **E.** meningitis

684. The frontal sinus is rarely involved with infection until the age of
- **A.** two to four years
- **B.** four to six years
- **C.** ten to 12 years
- **D.** 20 years
- **E.** six to ten years

685. Which of the following forms of sinusitis is associated with pain in the region of the temples and over the eyes?
- **A.** Sphenoid
- **B.** Frontal
- **C.** Anterior ethmoid
- **D.** Maxillary
- **E.** Mastoid

686. Sinobronchitis may be seen in association with all of the following EXCEPT
  A. chronic sinusitis
  B. cystic fibrosis
  C. α1-antitrypsin deficiency
  D. patients with allergy who smoke
  E. chronic use of vasoconstrictive nose drops for vasomotor rhinitis

687. Indications for tonsillectomy include all of the following EXCEPT
  A. peritonsillar abscess
  B. symptomatic hypertrophy
  C. suppurative cervical adenitis
  D. acute or chronic sinusitis
  E. repeated Group A strep infection in patients with rheumatic fever receiving strep prophylaxis

688. The most common complication of tonsillectomy is
  A. infection
  B. obstruction
  C. bleeding
  D. hoarseness
  E. serous otitis media

689. Which of the following statements concerning juvenile papilloma is FALSE?
  A. It is the most common benign tumor of the larynx in children
  B. It usually grows from vocal cords
  C. It often disappears after age 12 years
  D. The first symptom is hoarseness
  E. It usually disappears by age four years

690. All of the following may be associated with bronchial foreign bodies EXCEPT
  A. differences in valvular mechanisms are responsible in large part for the clinical symptoms
  B. fluoroscopic examination is invaluable as a diagnostic aid
  C. a high percentage of foreign bodies will be spontaneously removed by coughing
  D. secondary infection may occur if removal is delayed
  E. direct visualization by bronchoscopy and removal are commonly employed

691. Infectious croup may be associated with all of the following EXCEPT
A. parainfluenza virus
B. *H. influenzae*
C. a family history of croup in 15% of cases, and a history of recurrent laryngitis in the patient
D. airway obstruction severe enough to require assisted ventilation
E. permanent loss of hearing

692. Acute epiglottitis can occur in patients with all of the following EXCEPT
A. viral infections
B. acute onset of severe and progressive airway obstruction
C. hyperextension of neck
D. *H. influenzae* infection
E. *E. coli* infection

693. In contrast to acute epiglottitis, acute laryngotracheobronchitis has all of the following features EXCEPT
A. a more insidious onset
B. the etiologic agent is almost always viral
C. a slower course
D. the etiologic agent is almost always bacterial
E. the patient is less likely to require intubation

694. Which of the following would NOT be included in the differential diagnosis of acute infectious croup?
A. Diphtheria
B. Foreign body inhalation
C. Parainfluenza viral infection
D. Retropharyngeal abscess
E. Laryngeal papilloma

695. Which of the following statements concerning the management of croup syndrome is true?
A. All patients should be hospitalized immediately
B. X-rays are usually unrewarding
C. Antibiotics are always indicated
D. Tracheostomy is employed in most cases
E. The majority of patients do not require hospitalization

696. Which of the following statements concerning acute bronchitis is FALSE?
    A. It is usually viral in origin
    B. May culture organisms of known pathogenicity from sputum with good correlation with response to therapy
    C. It usually occurs as an isolated clinical entity in children
    D. Vomiting is frequently part of the clinical picture
    E. Increased fluid intake is advisable

697. Pneumococcal pneumonia is associated with all of the following EXCEPT
    A. it is the most common form of bacterial pneumonia in children
    B. serotypes causing disease in children differ from those of adults
    C. type-specific antibody will provide protection from reinfection
    D. prevention by pneumococcal vaccine may be possible in older children
    E. sickle cell anemia (SS) patients have no demonstrated increased risk factor for this infection

698. Concerning the symptoms of pneumococcal pneumonia in childhood, all of the following are true EXCEPT
    A. infants may be free of rales early in the course
    B. meningismus is not uncommon
    C. classic symptoms of consolidation are noted on either the second or third day of illness
    D. most patients do not give history of URI
    E. pneumococcal vaccine may not prove to serve as effective prophylaxis in infants under one year of age

699. The WBC and differential seen most often in patients with pneumococcal pneumonia are
    A. 10,000 mm^3 with left shift
    B. 20,000 mm^3 with right shift
    C. 5,000 mm^3 with marked left shift
    D. 10,000 mm^3 with right shift
    E. 15,000 to 40,000 mm^3 with left shift

700. Which of the following statements is true concerning staphylococcal pneumonia?
  A. It is the most common cause of bacterial pneumonia in infants less than a year of age
  B. Penicillin G is the drug of choice to initiate therapy
  C. The case fatality rate is 40% to 60%
  D. Unilateral lung involvement is most common
  E. It is the most common cause of pneumonia in sickle cell patients

701. Kartagener's syndrome includes all of the following EXCEPT
  A. occurrence in older patients
  B. presence of complete situs inversus
  C. paranasal sinusitis and bronchiectasis are present
  D. it is a treatable condition, in part
  E. it is always apparent in first year of life

DIRECTIONS: For each of the questions or incomplete statements below, **ONE** or **MORE** of the answers or completions given is correct. Select
  A if only *1, 2 and 3* are correct,
  B if only *1 and 3* are correct,
  C if only *2 and 4* are correct,
  D if only *4* is correct,
  E if all are correct.

---

702. Stridor in the newborn may be caused by
  1. laryngomalacia
  2. laryngeal web
  3. laryngeal paralysis secondary to trauma
  4. laryngeal papillomas

703. In the respiratory tract, mycoplasma can produce
  1. pharyngotonsillitis
  2. otitis media
  3. pneumonia
  4. pulmonary abscess

Directions Summarized				
A	B	C	D	E
1,2,3	1,3	2,4	4	All are
only	only	only	only	correct

704. In patients with cystic fibrosis
1. there is always positive family history
2. the earliest pulmonary symptoms may be coughing
3. bronchopleural fistulas are common
4. cor pulmonale may develop

705. Etiologic agents involved in acute pharyngitis include
1. *C. diphtheriae*
2. *Streptococcus pyogenes*
3. Coxsackie virus
4. *S. aureus*

706. Diseases that mainly affect the pulmonary interstitium include
1. sarcoidosis
2. hypersensitivity lung disease
3. pulmonary hemosiderosis
4. systemic lupus erythematosus with pulmonary involvement

707. In the development of the paranasal sinuses
1. maxillary antrum is present at birth
2. the frontal sinuses are present at birth
3. the sphenoidal sinuses are present at birth
4. the maxillary sinuses are present at birth

708. In regard to familial pectus excavatum
1. it is a common feature in congenital heart disease
2. surgical repair is indicated
3. lung capacity is usually decreased by 15%
4. it is rarely, if ever, a cause of pulmonary disability

709. Indications for tonsillectomy include
1. frequent respiratory infections
2. symptomatic hypertrophy
3. chronic otitis media
4. chronic tonsillar infection

710. In congenital diaphragmatic hernia
   1. the diagnosis may be sugested by ausculting bowel sounds in the thorax
   2. pulmonary hypoplasia is common
   3. surgery is indicated
   4. mechanical ventilation has not increased survival

711. Nasal polyps are frequently associated with
   1. allergic rhinitis
   2. acute leukemia
   3. cystic fibrosis
   4. chronic nose-picking

XIV: Respiratory System
Answers and Comments

653. D. Diabetes mellitus has been reported to have developed only in cystic fibrosis patients surviving into the late second and third decades of life. *(REF. 1 — p. 993)*

654. E. Twenty-five percent of CF patients will have some degree of cirrhosis at autopsy. *(REF. 1 — p. 993)*

655. A. The mode of inheritance of cystic fibrosis is autosomal recessive, with incidence estimated at one per 1,000 to one per 4,000 fetuses in the Caucasian population. *(REF. 1 — p. 993)*

656. E. Lack of pancreatic lipase is the explanation for failure of pyloric closure through neuronal mediation. Carbohydrate absorption is usually normal. *(REF. 1 — p. 994)*

657. E. The normal level is 5 to 50 mEq/L. Siblings and parents sometimes show modest elevations. *(REF. 1 — p. 995)*

658. E. There are occasional reports of the disease occurring without abnormal sweat electrolytes. *(REF. 1 — p. 995)*

659. A. Fat is the least tolerated, and a high-protein and high-carbohydrate diet is recommended. *(REF. 1 — p. 996)*

660. E. Complete correction is rarely achieved with any single mode of therapy, but improvement is noted in most patients with use of medium-chain triglyceride oil, enzyme therapy and reduction of long-chain fats in diet. *(REF. 1 — p. 996)*

661. E. The nasal passage will also warm inspired air to nearly that of the body's temperature. *(REF. 3 — p. 935)*

662. A. Those with only one side affected may be asymptomatic at birth; most with bilateral involvement have severe symptoms. *(REF. 2 — p. 1170)*

663. B. Surgery may be delayed for weeks, months, or years in patients with oral breathing. *(REF. 2 — p. 1170)*

664. E. Obstruction may well be followed by malodorous purulent discharge. *(REF. 2 — p. 1171)*

665. A. Trauma, especially nose-picking, is the most common cause. *(REF. 2 — p. 1171)*

666. C. In addition to showing up in the vomitus, blood that is swallowed during a nosebleed at night may also be found in the stool. *(REF. 2 — p. 1171)*

667. C. These two agents are responsible for the great majority of respiratory infections. *(REF. 2 — p. 1172)*

668. A. Staphylococcal organisms may be recovered by culture but do not cause primary disease in this location. *(REF. 2 — p. 1172)*

669. E. RSV is the most important respiratory tract pathogen found in the first two to three years of life. *(REF. 2 — p. 1172)*

670. D. Parainfluenza virus causes the majority of cases of croup syndrome but also is the cause of bronchitis and URI. *(REF. 2 — p. 1172)*

671. A. Except during epidemics, influenza viruses are rarely agents of respiratory syndromes in infants and children. Most influenza virus disease in infants and children involve the upper respiratory tract. *(REF. 2 — p. 1172)*

672. D. Primarily infection peaks in the second and third decades of life. *(REF. 2 — p. 1172)*

673. E. Rhinovirus will produce cold symptoms in at least 50% of susceptible patients. *(REF. 2 — p. 905)*

674. C. The number of exposures appears to be more important than any other single factor. *(REF. 3 — p. 940)*

675. E. Some normal children may have more than three to six colds per year. The infection is most common at two to three years of age. *(REF. 3 — p. 940)*

676. C. Otitis media occurs most commonly in infants and can be expected if fever recurs. *(REF. 2 — p. 906)*

677. E. Nasal obstruction can usually be controlled with judicious use of vasoconstricting nose drops. *(REF. 3 — p. 941)*

678. E. Little evidence exists to support the mucosal-shrinking effects of these agents even though they are widely prescribed. Drug side effects include sedation and excitation. *(REF. 3 — p. 941)*

679. E. In epidemics, strep may account for many more cases. *(REF. 3 — p. 942)*

680. B. A petechial follicular rash on the soft palate is another finding more often associated with strep than other infectious agents. *(REF. 2 — pp. 737–738)*

681. C. This high percentage of carriers may make diagnosis in sick children difficult. *(REF. 2 — p. 737)*

682. A. In adenoviral pharyngitis, the most striking finding is follicular injection of bulbar and palpebral conjunctiva. *(REF. 2 — pp. 903–905)*

683. C. These nodes drain portions of the nasopharynx and posterior nasal passages. *(REF. 2 — p. 1173)*

684. E. Pneumatization may be demonstrable by age two to four years, although infection does not occur until six to ten years of age. The development of the frontal sinuses may be delayed by severe ethmoid infection. *(REF. 2 — pp. 1174–1175)*

685. C. In posterior ethmoidal sinusitis, pain is in the distribution of the trigeminal nerve, especially over the mastoid. *(REF. 2 — p. 1175)*

686. E. The use of vasoconstrictor nose drops may well cause rebound rhinitis but it is not a known etiology for the sinobronchitis syndrome. *(REF. 2 — pp. 1175–1176)*

687. D. Tonsillectomy would be of no value either in the treatment or prevention of sinusitis. *(REF. 2 — p. 1178)*

688. C. Bleeding may be difficult to stop, requiring packing or ligation. *(REF. 2 — p. 1179)*

689. E. There is a high rate of recurrence with these lesions after surgical removal. Often after age 12 the lesions do not recur. *(REF. 2 — p. 1201)*

690. C. Only 2% to 4% of foreign bodies are coughed up. *(REF. 2 — pp. 1197–1200)*

691. E. All of the statements are true concerning infectious croup except permanent hearing loss, which has not been described. *(REF. 2 — p. 1193)*

692. E. Acute epiglottitis is not associated with *E. coli* organisms, which have not been identified as an etiology. *(REF. 2 — pp. 1193–1194)*

693. D. All of the statements concerning laryngotracheobronchitis are true except D. The etiologic agent is usually viral and contrasts vividly with epiglottitis, which is usually a rapidly progressing hemophilus infection with abrupt onset. *(REF. 2 — p. 1194)*

694. E. With benefit of adequate history, laryngeal papilloma would not be included because of the presence of hoarseness weeks before airway obstruction becomes a problem; all of the other etiologies are possibilities, with viral etiology the most common. *(REF. 2 — pp. 1193–1195)*

695. E. All of the other statements are incorrect. Many patients with the syndrome may be managed at home, and antibiotics are usually reserved for suspected bacterial infections. X-rays, especially fluoroscopic studies, can be most valuable in the differential diagnosis. *(REF. 2 — pp. 1195–1196)*

696. C. In children, bronchitis usually occurs in association with infection of the upper respiratory tract and the trachea. *(REF. 2 — p. 1202)*

697. E. All of the above statements are true except E. Sickle cell anemia patients are at increased risk for pneumococcal infection. *(REF. 2 — pp. 1207–1208)*

698. D. Most patients do describe a brief upper respiratory infection. *(REF. 2 — p. 1208)*

699. E. The usual WBC and differential are in the range of 15,000 to 40,000 with a preponderance of polymorphonuclear cells. *(REF. 2 — p. 1208)*

700. D. Unilateral involvement occurs in the right lung in about 65% of cases; bilateral involvement, in less than 20% of patients. *(REF. 2 — p. 1210)*

701. E. This is a symptom complex seen only in older patients. *(REF. 2 — p. 1293)*

702. E. All of the choices listed can be the cause of stridor in the newborn infant. *(REF. 1 — p. 1554)*

703. A. Mycoplasma can produce pharyngotonsillitis, otitis media, and pneumonia, with or without pleural effusion. It is not associated with pulmonary abscess. *(REF. 2 — p. 1172)*

704. C. The earliest symptom of cystic fibrosis may be cough. Cor pulmonale is a late finding in CF, after pulmonary fibrosis has occurred and pulmonary hypertension has become severe. Bronchopleural fistulae are rare complications. Most cases of CF are sporadic, representing spontaneous mutations. *(REF. 1 — p. 1565)*

705. A. *C. diphtheriae, S. pyogenes,* and Coxsackie virus all are causes of acute pharyngitis. *S. aureus* is not considered a pharyngeal pathogen. *(REF. 2 — pp. 737, 748, 919)*

706. E. All of the items listed involve pathology of the pulmonary interstitium. *(REF. 1 — p. 1584)*

707. B. Only the maxillary antrum and the sphenoidal sinuses are present at birth. *(REF. 2 — pp. 1169–1170)*

708. D. Pectus excavatum is rarely, if ever, a cause of pulmonary disability nor is it a common feature of CHD. Surgery is not indicated. *(REF. 1 — p. 1592)*

709. C. Of those listed, the only indications for tonsillectomy are symptomatic hypertrophy and chronically infected tonsils. *(REF. 2 — p. 1178)*

710. A. In congenital diaphragmatic hernia the diagnosis may be suggested by ausculating bowel sounds in the chest. Surgery is absolutely indicated, and mechanical ventilation increases the chances of survival tremendously. Pulmonary hypoplasia is common. *(REF. 1 — p. 1542)*

711. B. Nasal polyps are most frequently associated with allergic rhinitis and cystic fibrosis. *(REF. 2 — p. 1177)*

XV: Gastrointestinal System

DIRECTIONS: Each of the questions or incomplete statements below is followed by five suggested answers or completions. Select the **one** that is **BEST** in each case.

---

712. The minimal amount of blood loss usually necessary to produce gross change in stool appearance in children is
    A. 10 ml/day
    B. 2 ml/day
    C. 20 ml/day
    D. 5 ml/day
    E. 8 ml/day

713. A flat postabsorptive blood sugar curve can be observed in diarrheal states because of all of the following EXCEPT
    A. defects of absorption
    B. increased gut motility
    C. delayed gastric emptying
    D. defects of digestion
    E. disturbance of renal function

714. The minimal fluid intake recommended for a six-month-old infant with mild diarrhea is
    A. 300 ml/kg/24 hr
    B. 75 ml/kg/24 hr
    C. 150 ml/kg/24 hr
    D. 50 ml/kg/24 hr
    E. 500 ml/kg/24 hr

715. Which of the following is NOT a common finding at autopsy in a patient who suffered with severe diarrhea?
A. Fatty liver
B. Thrombosis of cerebral venous sinuses
C. Cerebral hemorrhages
D. Retinal hemorrhages
E. Gastric ulcers

716. Light microscopy of intestinal mucosa lesions in celiac disease shows
A. enlargement of villi
B. a reduction in the monocellular population of the lamina propria
C. ulcerations
D. loss of villi
E. increased length of microvilli

717. Intolerance to what nutrient source has the closest association to exacerbations in the patient with idiopathic celiac disease?
A. Starch
B. Butterfat
C. Wheat flour
D. Fructose
E. Glucose

718. The symptoms of celiac disease usually begin at
A. six to 12 months
B. five to six years
C. eight to ten years
D. three to four years
E. ten to 12 years

719. The fundamental defect in celiac disease is malabsorption of
A. fat
B. protein
C. disaccharides
D. starch
E. monosaccharides

720. The latent period of idiopathic celiac disease occurs in
    A. the first and second years of life
    B. the second and third years of life
    C. the fifth and sixth years of life
    D. late childhood and adolescence
    E. the third decade of life

721. What percentage of fat do children with celiac disease generally absorb from their diets?
    A. 50 to 60
    B. 75 to 85
    C. 40 to 50
    D. 0 to 10
    E. 30 to 40

722. In the patient with celiac disease and demonstrated gluten sensitivity, all of the following would be eliminated from the diet EXCEPT
    A. wheat
    B. rye
    C. oats
    D. barley
    E. rice

723. The patient with glucose-galactose malabsorption has all of the following EXCEPT
    A. normal intestinal disaccharide activity
    B. glycosuria
    C. severe, watery diarrhea on ingestion of glucose
    D. constipation
    E. severe, watery diarrhea with milk ingestion

724. The best method of diagnosing disaccharide malabsorption is
    A. family history
    B. biopsy and direct assay
    C. tolerance tests utilizing blood sugar assay
    D. stool pH
    E. reducing substances positive in stool

725. Protein-losing gastroenteropathy has been associated with all
of the following EXCEPT
A. cow milk protein
B. lymphangiectasia
C. granulomatous disease of intestine
D. ulcerative colitis
E. soy protein formula

726. Which of the following statements regarding the stools of a
child with an irritable colon syndrome is FALSE?
A. They number three to ten per day
B. They usually are passed in the space of a few hours early
in the day
C. They often contain mucus
D. They frequently are bloody
E. They may contain particles of undigested food, such as
corn kernels

727. Irritable colon syndrome in children is associated with
A. steatorrhea
B. protein malabsorption
C. growth failure
D. pathogenic bacteria in the stools
E. spontaneous remissions

728. The clinical features of milk-associated gastroenteropathy in-
clude all of the following EXCEPT
A. iron-deficiency anemia
B. positive guaiac tests
C. tolerance to skim milk
D. protein loss in the stool
E. diarrhea

729. The treatment for irritable colon syndrome in a two-year-old
child is a
A. low-fat diet
B. milk-free diet
C. low-residue diet
D. low-carbohydrate diet
E. normal diet for age

730. Organic causes for the symptom of chronic abdominal pain include all of the following EXCEPT
    A. constipation
    B. regional enteritis
    C. urinary tract infection
    D. chronic appendicitis
    E. ulcerative colitis

731. The major organic cause for recurrent abdominal pain in children is
    A. peptic ulcer
    B. regional enteritis
    C. Meckel's diverticulum
    D. urinary tract disease
    E. Hirshsprung's disease

732. The most useful clinical tool for differentiating congenital aganglionosis from functional constipation is
    A. early onset of symptoms
    B. marked infrequency of stools
    C. appearance of stools
    D. absence of urge to defecate
    E. response to laxative therapy

733. All of the following are useful in the management of chronic constipation EXCEPT
    A. mineral oil
    B. reduction of milk in diet
    C. increase in dietary fiber
    D. once weekly bowel evacuation by enema
    E. regular use of natural laxative foods

734. Anal pruritus occurring mainly at night is most often associated with
    A. encopresis
    B. hemorrhoids
    C. pinworms
    D. roundworms
    E. hookworms

735. The most common type of congenital esophageal malformation is
    A. esophageal atresia with distal tracheoesophageal fistula
    B. esophageal atresia without fistula
    C. tracheoesophageal fistula without atresia
    D. esophageal atresia with proximal tracheoesophageal fistula
    E. esophageal atresia, and proximal and distal tracheoesophageal fistula

736. An infant with the most common type of congenital esophageal malformation will present with all of the following symptoms EXCEPT
    A. coughing
    B. choking with feedings
    C. excessive oral secretions
    D. gasless abdomen
    E. cyanosis associated with feedings

737. In live births, the incidence of congenital malformation of the esophagus is
    A. one in 1,000
    B. one in 20,000
    C. one in 10,000
    D. one in 4,000
    E. one in 100,000

738. Features common to all patients with regional enteritis include all of the following EXCEPT
    A. delayed growth
    B. abdominal pain and diarrhea
    C. onset in more than 80% by 21 years of age
    D. involvement of the terminal ileum in over 80% cases
    E. fever

739. Therapy directed at patients with regional enteritis should include
    A. early surgical intervention via resection of gut with disease
    B. megavitamin therapy
    C. corticosteroid therapy
    D. routine high-dose potassium supplementation
    E. high-fiber diet

740. Which of the following features is NOT part of the clinical course in the patient with ulcerative colitis?
    A. Diarrhea and abdominal pain are the most common presenting features
    B. Barium enema is always diagnostic at the onset of symptoms
    C. Anemia is common
    D. Liver disease is an uncommon complication in children
    E. Colectomy

741. The symptom less frequently encountered in patients with regional enteritis vs patients with ulcerative colitis is
    A. rectal bleeding
    B. abdominal pain
    C. anemia
    D. diarrhea
    E. weight loss

742. Children presenting with peritonitis usually exhibit all of the following EXCEPT
    A. obscure symptomatology
    B. polymorphonuclear leukocytosis of 10,000–25,000 cells/mm^3
    C. *E. coli* as the most common organism
    D. total neutrophil count less than 3,000 cells/mm^3
    E. fever

743. In the pediatric patient, perforation of the stomach is most likely to be seen
    A. in the first few days of life
    B. in association with total distal obstruction
    C. in the same patient as a recurrence
    D. as a demonstrable congenital deficiency of muscle fibers in the stomach wall
    E. in association with partial distal obstruction

744. All of the following are true concerning intussusception EXCEPT
    A. it usually affects infants in the first two years of life
    B. a local lesion is usually found as a cause
    C. most cases begin at or near the ileocecal valve
    D. males are more frequently affected than females
    E. it affects whites more often than blacks

745. The signs and symptoms of intussusception may include all of the following EXCEPT
    A. the infant is well nourished and hydrated
    B. attacks of colicky pain recurring regularly with intervals in which the infant is prostrated
    C. the presence of blood and mucus in stools
    D. vomiting occurs as the initial symptom in 50% of cases
    E. abdominal pain is presenting complaint in 90% of patients

746. Which of the following statements is true in regard to the treatment of intussusception?
    A. Treatment should be delayed for four to six hours owing to the high incidence of spontaneous reduction
    B. Recurrence is more common after hydrostatic pressure reduction than operative reduction
    C. Hydrostatic pressure reduction is the method of choice
    D. Distension is an absolute contraindication for hydrostatic pressure reduction
    E. Rupture of bowel is frequently a complication of hydrostatic pressure reduction

747. Rectal prolapse can be seen in children with all of the following EXCEPT
    A. cystic fibrosis
    B. severe malnutrition
    C. whooping cough
    D. phimosis
    E. pinworm infestation

748. Concerning benign polyps of the gastrointestinal tract, which of the following is FALSE?
    A. Most common intestinal tumor
    B. Usually occurs in the colon
    C. Most frequent symptom is bleeding
    D. Bleeding is usually profuse
    E. Blood is generally bright red

749. Which of the following is FALSE concerning lympho-sarcoma of the bowel in childhood?
    A. Most common malignant tumor of the bowel
    B. Terminal ileum is most common site
    C. Usually diagnosed early because of intestinal obstruction
    D. Bleeding is rare
    E. History of chronic intussusception may be obtained

750. All of the following statements are true concerning replacement of potassium losses in the patient with severe diarrhea EXCEPT
    A. concentration in administered fluid should not exceed 40 mEq/L
    B. renal function must be present
    C. potassium losses should be replaced within 12 hours
    D. potassium is lost almost exclusively from the ICF
    E. elevations of serum potassium are a contraindication to IV therapy with potassium-containing solutions

751. All of the following metabolic alterations can occur in pyloric stenosis EXCEPT
    A. hypokalemia
    B. hypochloremia
    C. decreased serum pH
    D. dehydration
    E. alkalosis

752. All of the following may be features of pyloric stenosis EXCEPT
    A. it is more common in males
    B. it usually becomes symptomatic in first month of life
    C. initially there is nonprojectile vomiting
    D. vomitus is bile-stained
    E. failure to thrive

753. Which of the following statements concerning congenital high intestinal obstructions is FALSE?
    A. Vomiting may be persistent if there is no feeding of the infant
    B. Polyhydramnios is a frequent accompaniment
    C. Meconium stools may be passed initially
    D. Vomitus is always bile stained
    E. Farber test has limited value

754. All of the following statements are true of intestinal occlusions present at birth EXCEPT
A. stenosis is more common than atresia
B. the ileum is the site of 50% of lesions
C. infants with Down's syndrome have an increased incidence of duodenal atresia
D. in about 15% of infants multiple intestinal occlusions occur
E. symptoms may or may not be present at birth

755. All of the following are true concerning Meckel's diverticulum EXCEPT
A. it occurs in 2% to 3% of all persons
B. mucosal lining may be gastric, and this is the type most likely to produce symptoms
C. symptoms most commonly occur in the first two years of life
D. mucosal lining may be gastric and ileal, or colonic and ileal
E. acute painful hemorrhage is the most common symptom

756. The absence of ganglion cells of the intramural and submucous plexuses of the colon may be manifest by all of the following EXCEPT
A. severe enterocolitis in the neonate
B. the lesion occurs in 90% of cases in an area of bowel 4 to 25 cm proximal to anus
C. a patient who fails to thrive
D. history of obstipation and abdominal distention from early infancy
E. large stools and fecal soiling are common symptoms in children more than five years of age

757. Which of the following statements concerning Type II Crigler-Najjar syndrome is FALSE?
A. Onset is from birth to 10 years
B. Kernicterus is common in newborn period
C. Autosomal dominant inheritance
D. Phenobarbital is effective
E. Survival to adulthood is the rule

758. Crigler-Najjar Syndrome Type I is characterized by all of the following EXCEPT
   A. onset at birth of jaundice
   B. kernicterus is rare
   C. autosomal recessive inheritance
   D. phenobarbital is ineffective
   E. no hemolysis is present

759. Which of the following is FALSE concerning Gilbert's disease?
   A. Unconjugated bilirubin less than 6.2 mg/dl
   B. Onset before age 1 year
   C. Males 4.2:1 over females
   D. Phenobarbital effective
   E. Inheritance is autosomal dominant

760. Approximately what percentage of newborns with persistent jaundice and passage of acholic stools have hepatitis?
   A. 30
   B. 60
   C. 90
   D. 10
   E. 3

761. A deficiency of which of the following vitamins is suggestive evidence of biliary atresia in the infant with persistent jaundice and acholic stools?
   A. E
   B. C
   C. Thiamine
   D. Niacin
   E. B_{12}

762. The number of reported cases of infectious hepatitis in the U.S. each year is
   A. 2,000 to 4,000
   B. 10,000 to 20,000
   C. 50,000 to 70,000
   D. 100,000 to 200,000
   E. 30,000 to 50,000

763. Australia antigen is a marker associated with
    A. infectious hepatitis
    B. serum hepatitis
    C. hepatitis of any viral etiology
    D. alcoholic hepatitis
    E. α1-antitrypsin deficiency

764. What percentage of patients with neonatal hepatitis recover completely?
    A. 33%
    B. 66%
    C. 99%
    D. 10%
    E. Less than 2%

765. The incubation period for infectious hepatitis prior to onset of jaundice is
    A. 14 to 40 days
    B. 60 to 160 days
    C. 30 to 90 days
    D. two to three days
    E. 160 to 210 days

766. All of the following are symptoms characteristic of the early phase of infectious hepatitis EXCEPT
    A. fever
    B. malaise
    C. anorexia
    D. jaundice
    E. nausea and vomiting

767. Prednisone may be indicated in a patient with acute viral hepatitis for all the following reasons EXCEPT
    A. coma
    B. severe bleeding
    C. persistent fever
    D. jaundice of two weeks duration
    E. excessively abnormal blood chemistry values

768. Which of the major nutrients is less likely to have decreased absorption during diarrhea?
   A. Fat
   B. Monosaccharides
   C. Protein
   D. Starch
   E. Disaccharides

DIRECTIONS: Each group of questions below consists of five lettered headings followed by a list of numbered words, phrases or statements. For **each** numbered word, phrase or statement, select the **one** lettered heading that is most closely associated with it. Each lettered heading may be selected once, more than once, or not at all.

   A. Esophageal atresia
   B. Pyloric stenosis
   C. Chalasia
   D. Duodenal atresia
   E. Intussusception

769. High incidence in Down's syndrome

770. Bloody stool may be seen

771. Surgery is usually not indicated

772. Passage of radiopaque catheter is usually diagnostic

773. More frequent in male infants

774. Barium enema is indicated if there is no intestinal perforation

   A. Imperforate anus
   B. Celiac sprue
   C. Schwachman syndrome
   D. Intestinal lymphangectasia
   E. Acrodermatitis enteropathica

775. Associated with bone marrow failure

776. High incidence in Down's syndrome

777. Chronic diarrhea, alopecia, and dermatitis

778. Accompanied by an immune deficiency state

779. Second most common chronic malabsorption syndrome in children

780. Pancreatic exocrine insufficiency

    A. Alpha-1-fetoprotein
    B. Crigler-Najjar syndrome
    C. Reye's syndrome
    D. Wilson's disease
    E. Alpha-1-antitrypsin deficiency

781. Acute yellow atrophy of the liver and encephalopathy

782. Associated with the presence of hepatoblastoma

783. May present as neonatal hepatitis

784. Glucuronyl transferase deficiency

785. Associated involvement of the basal ganglia

786. May have emphysema in later life

XV: Gastrointestinal System
Answers and Comments

712. C. In children, blood losses up to about 15 ml/day may occur from any point in the intestinal tract without a gross change in appearance of stools. *(REF. 1 — p. 989)*

713. E. All of these factors except renal excretion defects would influence postprandial blood sugar curves. The only accurate method of measuring carbohydrate absorption is radioactive labeling. *(REF. 1 — p. 990)*

714. C. The minimum amount is 150 ml/kg/24 hr, and 300 ml/kg/24 hr would be unusual. *(REF. 1 — p. 991)*

715. E. The central nervous system pathology may contribute significantly to the mortality associated with diarrhea. Gastric ulcers would be the most rare finding. *(REF. 1 — p. 991)*

716. D. There is also loss of intervillous space. Electron micrographs reveal decreases and shortening of microvilli. *(REF. 1 — p. 998)*

717. C. A close correlation is observed between the ingestion of wheat flour and exacerbations. The disturbing factor in wheat lies in a protein moiety, gluten, particularly its gliadin component. *(REF. 1 — p. 998)*

718. A. It is rare for presentation before six months or after three years. *(REF. 1 — p. 999)*

719. A. Fat is the principal nutrient that is malabsorbed. The unabsorbed fecal fats are mainly the longer-chain saturated fatty acids. *(REF. 1 — p. 999)*

720. D. Even without treatment most patients will experience a marked decrease in symptomatology in late childhood and early adolescence. *(REF. 1 — p. 1000)*

721. D. Less than 90% of ingested fat is absorbed, with stool losses of 3 to 5 gm/day. *(REF. 1 — p. 1000)*

722. E. Strict adherence to this elimination diet usually results in complete freedom from symptoms. Rice does not cause symptoms. *(REF. 1 — p. 1000)*

723. D. Glycosuria is a common finding. Acquired malabsorption has been described in patients with surgical resections and acute episodes of gastroenteritis. Milk causes diarrhea because intestinal lactase breaks milk sugar down into glucose and galactose. *(REF. 1 — p. 1002)*

724. B. Biopsy of mucosa of small intestine and direct assay of disaccharides are the best methods. *(REF. 1 — pp. 1004, 1005)*

725. E. These children will suffer from edema and will demonstrate hypoproteinemia without proteinuria. Protein-losing gastroenteropathy has not been described in association with soy protein ingestion. *(REF. 1 — p. 1006)*

726. D. This syndrome usually begins at about six months and ceases between three or four years of age. Blood is not detectable in the stool. *(REF. 1 — p. 1007)*

727. E. These children grow normally despite recurrent bouts of loose stools. Spontaneous remissions at age three to four years are the rule. *(REF. 1 — p. 1007)*

728. C. It is the protein of cow's milk to which the patients are intolerant. *(REF. 1 — p. 1007)*

729. E. Dietary modifications are unnecessary, are potentially harmful, and lead to nutritionally unbalanced diets and needless parental concern. Some advocate avoidance of iced foods for children with irritable colon syndrome. *(REF. 1 — pp. 1007, 1008)*

730. D. Chronic appendicitis and chronic mesenteric lymphadenitis are diagnoses in considerable doubt in modern pediatrics. *(REF. 1 — p. 1010)*

731. D. Every patient with the complaint of recurrent abdominal pain deserves urinalysis. *(REF. 1 — p. 1010)*

732. D. The proprioceptors that initiate the reflex urge to defecate are located just proximal to the internal sphincter and are rarely activated in the patient with Hirschsprung's disease. *(REF. 1 — p. 1012)*

733. D. Behavior modification with reward for regular attempts at stooling will be valuable also. Enemas should not be a regular part of a therapy plan. They may be useful in the initial stages of a therapy program. *(REF. 1 — pp. 1012, 1013)*

734. C. Other causes of pruritus ani cause symptoms day and night. Roundworms and hookworms are not associated with anal itching. *(REF. 1 — p. 1014)*

735. A. This variety accounts for about 86% of all cases. *(REF. 1 — p. 1015)*

736. D. The distal tracheoesophageal fistula allows large quantities of air into the gastrointestinal tract. *(REF. 1 — p. 1015)*

737. D. One in 4,000 live births will have a deformity involving atresia and fistula, or rarely atresia alone. *(REF. 1 — p. 1015)*

738. C. Onset of illness has been reported to be 10% to 15% by age 15 years; about half experience onset by 21 years. *(REF. 1 — pp. 1046, 1047)*

739. C. Corticosteroid therapy is eventually required for most patients and is useful in control of the disease. Megavitamin therapy is of no proved benefit. Surgical intervention is restricted to specific complications. *(REF. 1 — pp. 1046, 1047)*

740. B. Barium enema may appear entirely normal for periods up to two to three years after onset of disease. *(REF. 1 — p. 1049)*

741. A. The diarrhea of regional enteritis is rarely bloody and rectal bleeding has not been observed. *(REF. 1 — pp. 1046–1051)*

742. D. All of the other statements are true; older children, like adults, usually have well-marked and characteristic symptoms. A polymorphonuclear leukocytosis of 10,000 to 25,000 cells/mm^3 is almost always present. Only in the most severely ill patients with sepsis is neutropenia observed. *(REF. 1 — p. 1053)*

743. A. The lesion is almost exclusively seen in this age group and rarely is it associated with distal obstructive lesions of either the total or partial variety. *(REF. 1 — p. 1056)*

744. B. A cause is rarely clear. In only 2.5% of cases under two years of age is a cause identifiable. *(REF. 1 — p. 1057)*

745. E. Abdominal pain as the initial symptom occurs in about 50% of patients, which is about the same frequency as with vomiting as the initial complaint. *(REF. 1 — p. 1058)*

746. C. Hydrostatic pressure reduction is the method of choice because discomfort is less than that with surgery. The complications in the absence of anesthesia are fewer, and the period of hospitalization is much shorter. *(REF. 1 — p. 1059)*

747. E. All of these conditions except pinworms have been associated with rectal prolapse. Recurrent episodes are most commonly seen in patients with cystic fibrosis. Any condition that increases the intra-abdominal pressure may precipitate prolapse, and malnutrition may be a significant contributing factor. *(REF. 1 — pp. 1059, 1060)*

748. D. Rarely is bleeding from benign polyps profuse. The blood may be mixed with the stool or be present on the surface of the stool. *(REF. 1 — p. 1061)*

749. C. The tumor is usually diagnosed quite late owing to its insidious infiltration, which eventually leads to intestinal obstruction. *(REF. 1 — p. 1062)*

750. C. Potassium losses should be replaced over a three-to-four-day period. *(REF. 2 — p. 270)*

751. C. Pyloric stenosis usually results in hypochloremic alkalosis. This can be corrected by the administration of fluids containing sodium and potassium. *(REF. 2 — p. 296)*

752. D. The vomitus is not bile-stained in pyloric stenosis. *(REF. 2 — p. 1051)*

753. D. The vomitus will contain bile if the obstruction is below the ampulla of Vater as is usually, but not always, the case. *(REF. 2 — p. 1053)*

754. A. Atresia is the more common lesion. Symptoms may be delayed an indeterminate length of time if the obstruction is incomplete. *(REF. 2 — p. 1054)*

755. E. Bleeding is the most common symptom, but it is not accompanied by pain. Bleeding is usually acute, but may be intermittent and recurrent. *(REF. 2 — p. 1060)*

756. E. The stools of the older infant or child may have a consistency of small pellets or be ribbon-like or have a fluid consistency. Large stools and fecal soiling are typical of the patient with functional constipation. *(REF. 2 — p. 1057)*

757. B. Kernicterus does not occur in any age group and survival to adulthood is the rule. *(REF. 2 — pp. 1114, 1115)*

758. B. Kernicterus is usual, with death in infancy. There is no hemolytic process in either Type I or Type II Crigler-Najjar syndrome. *(REF. 2 — p. 1114)*

759. B. Onset is delayed to ten years or more in this autosomal dominantly inherited disease. There are often significant associated symptoms, such as fatigue, malaise and gastrointestinal complaints, in addition to jaundice. *(REF. 2 — p. 1115)*

760. A. Most of the others have atresia of the extrahepatic biliary tree. *(REF. 2 — p. 883)*

761. A. Vitamin E, a fat-soluble vitamin, is poorly absorbed when bile salts are absent from the intestinal tract and can be used as a diagnostic test. Patients do not necessarily show clinical symptoms of vitamin E deficiency. *(REF. 2 — pp. 883, 884)*

762. C. This probably represents no more than 10% of the actual number of cases, since a large number go undiagnosed because of lack of symptoms. *(REF. 2 — p. 907)*

763. B. Serum, or long-incubation Type B, hepatitis frequently contains this antigen. *(REF. 2 — p. 907)*

764. A. Two-thirds of patients will die or progress to postnecrotic cirrhosis. *(REF. 2 — p. 911)*

765. A. If measured from the onset of initial symptoms, it may be three to five days less. *(REF. 2 — p. 885)*

766. D. All the other symptoms usually occur four to five days before the onset of jaundice. *(REF. 2 — p. 909)*

767. D. Severe jaundice, whether it be of long or short duration, is an indicator for treatment with prednisone. Marked decreases in prothrombin time values may indicate need for prednisone therapy. *(REF. 2 — p. 887)*

768. C. Protein assimilation is affected relatively little. *(REF. 1 — p. 990)*

769. D. The diagnosis of intussusception is confirmed by barium
770. E. enema, and this procedure can be curative; it is therefore
771. C. indicated if perforation has not occurred. Bloody stool is
772. A. common. There is a high incidence of duodenal atresia in
773. B. Down's syndrome. Chalasia is not considered a surgical
774. E. problem. Pyloric stenosis is seen more commonly in males. Esophageal atresia can be diagnosed by the passage of a radiopaque catheter. *(REF. 2 — pp. 803–831)*

775. C. Schwachman's syndrome is pancreatic exocrine failure
776. A. with bone marrow failure. Celiac sprue is the second most
777. E. common chronic malabsorption syndrome in childhood.
778. D. Intestinal lymphangiectasia has an associated immune
779. B. deficiency. Acrodermatitis enteropathica is described as
780. C. chronic diarrhea, dermatitis of extremities and mucous membranes, and alopecia. There is a high incidence of imperforate anus in Down's syndrome. *(REF. 2 — pp. 850–861)*

781. C. In alpha-1-antitrypsin deficiency, patients may present
782. A. with neonatal hepatitis and may develop emphysema as
783. E. young adults. Crigler-Najjar syndrome has glucuronyl
784. B. transferase deficiency as its cause. Reye's syndrome con-
785. D. sists of acute yellow atrophy of the liver and encepha-
786. E. lopathy. Wilson's disease involvement of the basal ganglia is a manifestation of its CNS lesion. Alpha-1-fetoprotein is associated with hepatoblastoma. *(REF. 2 — pp. 876–894)*

XVI: Blood and Blood-Forming Tissues

DIRECTIONS: Each of the questions or incomplete statements below is followed by five suggested answers or completions. Select the **one** that is **BEST** in each case.

---

787. During which month of gestation does hematopoiesis in the bone marrow begin?
    A. Third
    B. Fifth
    C. Sixth
    D. Seventh
    E. Eighth

788. In which of the following organs is erythropoietin primarily produced?
    A. Bone marrow
    B. Liver
    C. Kidney
    D. Spleen
    E. Intestines

789. Which of the following globin chain combinations is present in hemoglobin F?
    A. Alpha 2 gamma 2
    B. Alpha 2 beta 2
    C. Alpha 2 delta 2
    D. Alpha 2 epsilon 2
    E. Epsilon 4

790. Which of the following approximates the blood volume in older children?
    A. 90 ml/kg
    B. 85 ml/kg
    C. 80 ml/kg
    D. 75 ml/kg
    E. 70 ml/kg

791. A shift of the oxygen dissociation curve to the right (decreased affinity of the RBC for oxygen) is associated with all the following EXCEPT
    A. high altitude
    B. cyanosis
    C. anemia
    D. fetal life
    E. none of the above

792. A low mean corpuscular volume (MCV) in the face of anemia is associated with which of the following?
    A. Thalassemia minor
    B. Reticulocytosis
    C. Liver disease
    D. Chronic hypoplastic anemia
    E. Folate deficiency

793. A normal MCV and a normal reticulocyte index is usually associated with which of the following?
    A. Chronic disease
    B. Malignancy with bone marrow involvement
    C. Acute blood loss
    D. Acute aplastic anemia
    E. Malignancy without bone marrow involvement

794. Abnormalities associated with intravascular hemolysis include all of the following EXCEPT
    A. increase in plasma hemoglobin
    B. decrease in serum haptoglobin
    C. increase in urinary hemosiderin
    D. increase in serum unconjugated bilirubin
    E. none of the above

795. Which of the following is considered an excessively sensitive (sometimes false-positive) indicator of occult intestinal blood loss?
   A. Guaiac
   B. Benzidine reaction
   C. Rate of appearance of ^{59}Fe-labeled red cells in stool
   D. Rate of appearance of ^{131}I-labeled serum albumin in stool
   E. Rate of appearance of ^{51}Cr-labeled red cells in stool

796. Decreased red cell production is the cause of anemia due to a deficiency of all of the following EXCEPT
   A. vitamin E
   B. vitamin B_{12}
   C. iron
   D. folate
   E. none of the above

797. Under which of the following circumstances is iron absorption in the small intestine decreased?
   A. When it is complexed with fructose
   B. When it is complexed with ascorbic acid
   C. When it is complexed with histidine
   D. When it is complexed with lysine
   E. By formation of insoluble phosphates

798. In iron deficiency anemia, which of the following tests is LEAST reliable in determining the level of deficiency?
   A. Total serum iron
   B. Transferrin saturation
   C. Erythrocyte protoporphyrin level
   D. Serum iron-binding capacity
   E. Serum ferritin

799. With which of the following is a depressed serum ferritin (less than 7 ng/ml) more often associated?
   A. Chronic renal disease
   B. Rheumatoid arthritis
   C. Iron deficiency anemia
   D. Infection
   E. Malignancy

800. Which of the following is the single most useful aid to early diagnosis of folate deficiency?
   A. RBC indices
   B. Serum folate
   C. Hypersegmentation of neutrophil nuclei
   D. Bone marrow aspiration
   E. Whole blood folate

801. Juvenile pernicious anemia is characterized by all of the following EXCEPT
   A. gastric atrophy
   B. concurrent endocrinopathies
   C. selective IgA deficiency
   D. autosomal recessive inheritance pattern
   E. chronic candidiasis

802. Which of the following is NOT characteristic of congenital pernicious anemia?
   A. Autosomal recessive inheritance pattern
   B. Decreased secretion of normally active intrinsic factor
   C. Abnormal gastric mucosa
   D. No demonstrable antibodies
   E. No demonstrable associated endocrinopathies

803. Which of the following is the earliest clinical manifestation of vitamin B_{12} deficiency?
   A. Hypersegmented neutrophils
   B. Megaloblastic anemia
   C. Thrombocytopenia
   D. Mild jaundice
   E. Leukopenia

804. Copper deficiency is characterized by all of the following EXCEPT
   A. marked neutropenia
   B. loss of hair pigment
   C. cerebral degeneration
   D. megaloblastic anemia
   E. slow growth

805. Anemia of infection and chronic disease is associated with all of the following EXCEPT
   A. shortened red cell survival
   B. impaired utilization of iron
   C. normal amount of iron in erythroid precursors
   D. impaired erythropoietin and marrow response
   E. usually mild anemia with normocytic or microcytic red cells

806. Acquired aplastic anemia is commonly associated with all of the following EXCEPT
   A. hepatosplenomegaly
   B. purpura
   C. no characteristic morphologic abnormalities are evident on peripheral blood smear
   D. increase in the iron saturation of serum transferrin
   E. absence of adenopathy

807. Congenital aplastic anemia is commonly associated with all of the following EXCEPT
   A. hematologic manifestations appear after five years of age
   B. peripheral blood that reveals a macrocytic, normochromic anemia
   C. skeletal malformations of the upper extremities
   D. leukemia
   E. anemia is the usual presenting picture

808. Congenital hypoplastic anemia is usually characterized by all of the following EXCEPT
   A. it is clinically apparent by six months of age
   B. anemia is macrocytic and unaccompanied by abnormalities in white cell or platelet counts
   C. serum erythropoietin levels are depressed
   D. treatment with oral corticosteroid therapy will usually produce reticulocytosis within five to seven days
   E. lack of reticulocytosis

809. All of the following findings distinguish acquired hypoplastic anemia (transient erythroblastopenia) from congenital hypoplastic anemia EXCEPT
  A. it may have an early onset
  B. there is an absence of associated congenital anomalies
  C. red cells are not macrocytic and do not contain an increased percentage of fetal hemoglobin
  D. it may follow viral infections
  E. chronic steroid therapy is unnecessary

810. Which of the following Rh antigens is considered the most antigenic?
  A. C
  B. D
  C. E
  D. c
  E. e

811. Anti-D antibody (RhoGAM) should be administered to mothers under all the following circumstances EXCEPT
  A. Rh-negative mother not previously sensitized delivering a Rh-positive infant
  B. Rh-negative mother whose pregnancy has been terminated by an abortion
  C. mothers tested as Rh-negative but whose red cells contain the D^u allele
  D. Rh-negative mothers who deliver infants who are D^u antigen positive
  E. Rh-negative mother who has had an abortion prior to delivering an Rh-positive infant

812. Erythroblastosis fetalis is associated with all of the following EXCEPT
  A. fetal response to anemia with increased release of erythropoietin and increased hematopoiesis
  B. hepatic cellular necrosis in severe disease
  C. hypoinsulinism
  D. fetal growth is usually normal
  E. appearance of pulmonary surfactant is low

813. In the acute transient form of acquired immune hemolytic anemia which of the following is FALSE?
A. Usual onset in first four years of life
B. In addition to anemia, reticulocytopenia, thrombocytopenia, and neutropenia are usually present
C. Prognosis for the acute idiopathic transient form is good
D. Both direct and indirect Coombs' reactions are positive
E. Hemoglobinemia and hemoglobinuria may be observed

814. Which of the following is FALSE concerning drug-induced hemolytic anemia?
A. Drugs are rarely the cause of hemolysis in children
B. A positive Coombs' test may be found in patients receiving penicillin in high doses
C. Cephalothin commonly acts as a hapten, and in the ensuing reaction hemolytic anemia may develop
D. Alpha-methyldopa is the most common cause of drug-induced hemolytic anemia
E. The antibody formed against the combination of red cell membrane and penicillin is IgG

815. Paroxysmal nocturnal hemoglobinuria is characterized by all of the following EXCEPT
A. it is associated with a low plasma pH
B. other elements of the blood (WBC and platelets) are usually normal
C. major thrombotic episodes occasionally occur
D. the disease may terminate in leukemia
E. intravascular hemolysis

816. Which of the following statements is FALSE regarding the pathophysiology of sickle cell disease?
A. Infection is associated with increased anemia by suppression of RBC production
B. Conversion of RBC from normal biconcave discs to sickle forms require the deoxygenation of hemoglobin
C. Hypoxia and acidemia promote sickling by decreasing oxygen saturation of hemoglobin
D. Hypotonic dehydration promotes sickling
E. Sickle cells increase whole blood viscosity, producing local ischemia

817. Which of the following clinical manifestations is NOT common to sickle cell disease?
   A. Vaso-occlusive crisis is more common than aplastic crisis
   B. Hyperhemolytic crisis is often associated with red cell glucose-6-phosphate dehydrogenase (G6PD) deficiency
   C. Aplastic crisis is often associated with viral or bacterial infection
   D. Salmonella sepsis is commonly associated with salmonella osteomyelitis
   E. Hand-foot syndrome may be initial manifestation of sickle cell disease

818. Of the following organisms, which is most often associated with sepsis in sickle cell disease?
   A. Pneumococci
   B. *H. influenzae*
   C. *S. aureus*
   D. Salmonella
   E. Mycoplasma pneumonia

819. Sickle cell trait is usually characterized by all of the following EXCEPT
   A. red cell concentration of S hemoglobin is about 40%
   B. splenic infarcts rarely occur except under extreme hypoxic conditions
   C. reticulocyte count is usually mildly elevated
   D. in some individuals, hyposthenuria and hematuria may result from sickling in the renal medullary capillaries
   E. the incidence in American blacks is one in 12

820. Which of the following does NOT characterize heterozygous beta-thalassemia (minor or trait)?
   A. In most patients anemia and clinical symptoms are absent
   B. Life expectancy is shortened
   C. Varieties of this order are best distinguished by quantitation of A2 and F hemoglobins
   D. Peripheral blood examination reveals microcytosis, target cells, and variable degrees of hypochromia
   E. Severity depends on the degree of suppression of beta-globin synthesis

821. Beta-thalassemia major is associated with all of the following EXCEPT
   A. defect in β-globin chain synthesis
   B. the newborn infant is clinically and hematologically normal
   C. the determination of A2 hemoglobin is important in diagnosis
   D. onset of clinical signs and symptoms usually begins between six and 12 months of age
   E. peripheral blood shows hypochromic and usually microcytic anemia

822. In hereditary spherocytosis, all of the following are characteristic EXCEPT
   A. it is an autosomal dominant trait
   B. there is loss of red cell membrane surface area without a reduction of cell volume, necessitating a spherical shape in order to accommodate its contents
   C. spherocytes are more likely to rupture than normal cells when suspended in hypotonic solutions
   D. the MCV is increased and the mean corpuscular hemoglobin concentration (MCHC) is decreased
   E. clinical severity tends to be relatively consistent within families, although it varies widely from family to family

823. The characteristics most often observed in elliptocytosis include all of the following EXCEPT
   A. increased osmotic fragility of fresh erythrocytes
   B. hemolysis is well compensated, and reticulocytosis without significant anemia is noted
   C. elliptocytes may appear only gradually several months after birth
   D. splenectomy eliminates hemolysis in most patients with hemolytic forms of elliptocytosis
   E. no therapy is required for patients without hemolysis

824. Vitamin E deficiency is associated with all the following EXCEPT
   A. greater prevalence in small, premature infants
   B. manifestation as normocytic normochromic anemia with an elevated reticulocyte count
   C. acanthocytes are diagnostic
   D. the only physical manifestations characteristic of this deficiency are edema of legs, labia, and eyelids in infants
   E. it manifests itself as a mild hemolytic anemia

825. Characteristics of G6PD deficiency in patients include all of the following EXCEPT
   A. a sex-linked recessive pattern of inheritance
   B. persistence of low grade anemia in patients
   C. the most common clinical manifestation is episodic acute hemolysis usually following infection or drug ingestion
   D. in blacks, G6PD activity is near normal in reticulocytes and young erythrocytes
   E. Heinz bodies are present only early in hemolytic episodes

826. Methemoglobinemia is associated with all of the following EXCEPT
   A. it is caused by oxidation of heme iron to ferric state
   B. newborns are less susceptible because hemoglobin F is less readily oxidized to methemoglobin than is hemoglobin A
   C. M hemoglobinopathy, a form of methemoglobinemia, does not respond to methylene blue therapy
   D. a presumptive diagnosis can be made when fresh blood that is chocolate-brown in color does not become red when aerated by mixing
   E. the discovery of clinical cyanosis is usually the first suggestion of methemoglobinemia

827. The phagocytic function of neutrophils is characterized by all of the following EXCEPT
    A. chemotaxis is dependent in part upon the activation of the complement system
    B. the most important opsonins, which are necessary for neutrophilic recognition of particles, are antibodies of the IgA class
    C. the killing of bacteria takes place through hydrolytic digestion and is facilitated, in part, by the action of antibacterial proteins, such as lactoferrin, found in cytoplasmic granules
    D. phagocytic functions take place primarily in tissues
    E. phagosomes are associated with degranulation

828. Which of the following leukocytes serves the specialized function of ingesting antigen-antibody complexes?
    A. Neutrophils
    B. Monocytes
    C. Eosinophils
    D. Basophils
    E. Lymphocytes

829. The Schwachman-Diamond syndrome (hereditary pancreatic insufficiency and bone marrow hypoplasia) is associated with all of the following EXCEPT
    A. abnormal sweat test
    B. neutropenia and anemia
    C. steatorrhea
    D. growth retardation
    E. thrombocytopenia

830. The Chédiak-Steinbrinck-Higashi syndrome is characterized by all of the following EXCEPT
    A. neutropenia, probably the result of increased destruction of granulocytes within the bone marrow
    B. striking giant lysosomal granules present in neutrophils
    C. inability of neutrophils to phagocytose and kill bacteria
    D. albinism, photophobia, and nystagmus
    E. autosomal recessive mode of inheritance

831. The most common combination of bacterial organisms associated with acute adenitis is
    A. β-hemolytic streptococci (BHS) and pneumococci
    B. *H. influenzae*, BHS
    C. staphylococci, BHS
    D. staphylococci, pneumococci
    E. *H. influenzae*, staphylococci

832. All of the following features distinguish juvenile from the adult variety of chronic myelocytic leukemia EXCEPT
    A. thrombocytopenia rather than thrombocytosis
    B. less marked leukocytosis
    C. absence of the Philadelphia chromosome
    D. better response to chemotherapy
    E. high percentage of monocytes with monocytic rather than granulocytic colony formation in vitro

833. Hodgkin's disease is characterized by all of the following EXCEPT
    A. it is rare before five years of age
    B. the most common first manifestation is painless, progressive enlargement of a lymph node
    C. involvement of axillary and cervical nodes are equal
    D. there is no characteristic abnormality of the blood
    E. Pel-Ebstein fever

834. Non-Hodgkin's lymphoma (formerly termed lymphosarcoma, reticulum cell sarcoma or giant follicular lymphoma) differs from Hodgkin's disease in all of the following EXCEPT
    A. in NHL, malignant cells appear more poorly undifferentiated
    B. NHL is three to four times more common
    C. dissemination occurs earlier and more often in NHL
    D. there is a greater female-to-male ratio in NHL
    E. therapy is less effective

835. NHL is typically manifested by all of the following EXCEPT
   A. development of diffuse bone marrow involvement is uncommon
   B. CNS involvement is relatively rare
   C. blood count is usually normal in absence of marrow involvement
   D. diagnosis depends on histopathology of primary tumor mass or regional nodes
   E. primary disease of the abdomen often presents as intussusception

836. What percentage of normal newborns will be found to have palpable spleens?
   A. 10%
   B. 15%
   C. 25%
   D. 30%
   E. 5%

837. Asplenism is associated with all of the following EXCEPT
   A. congenital absence occurs commonly with partial situs inversus
   B. fulminant infections occur most often in young children with infections due to *H. influenzae*
   C. it should be suspected in the presence of Howell-Jolly bodies on peripheral blood smear
   D. life-threatening infections are more commonly associated with sickle cell anemia than with postsplenectomy due to idiopathic thrombocytopenic purpura
   E. the risk of fulminant infection postsplenectomy never completely diminishes with age

838. Which of the following bleeding disorders is characterized as autosomal dominant?
   A. Von Willebrand's disease
   B. Factor VIII deficiency
   C. Factor IX deficiency
   D. Factor VII deficiency
   E. Factor V deficiency

839. The prothrombin time (PT) is a function of all of the following EXCEPT
   A. factor II
   B. factor V
   C. factor VII
   D. factor X
   E. factor IX

840. Partial thrombosplastin time (PTT) is a function of all of the following EXCEPT
   A. factor VIII
   B. factor VII
   C. factor X
   D. factor XI
   E. factor IX

841. Vitamin K-dependent factors include all of the following clotting factors EXCEPT
   A. XI
   B. IX
   C. VII
   D. X
   E. II

842. In addition to the bleeding time, which of the following is also abnormal in von Willebrand's disease?
   A. Platelet count
   B. PTT
   C. Prothrombin time
   D. Thrombin time
   E. Factor VII level

843. Anaphylactoid purpura is manifested by all of the following EXCEPT
   A. urticarial lesions progressing to red maculopapular eruption
   B. polyarthritis due to intra-articular bleeding
   C. recurrent colicky abdominal pain due to edema and hemorrhage into intestinal wall
   D. renal involvement manifested by microscopic hematuria
   E. melena may be common

844. Which of the following laboratory findings is NOT characteristic of Henoch-Schönlein syndrome (anaphylactoid purpura)?
A. Thrombocytopenia
B. Proteinuria
C. Anemia
D. Normal hemostatic function
E. Leukocytosis

845. Idiopathic thrombocytopenic purpura (ITP) is characterized by all of the following EXCEPT
A. it is associated with antiplatelet antibody
B. it frequently follows viral infection in children
C. spontaneous remission is achieved in great majority of cases
D. prominent physical findings of splenomegaly are present
E. bone marrow examination may reveal increased platelet production

846. Which of the following laboratory findings is NOT characteristic of ITP?
A. Platelet count below $50,000/mm^3$
B. Normal PT, PTT, normal thrombin time (TT)
C. Normal WBC
D. Bone marrow reveals decreased number of megakaryocytes
E. Clotting retraction is poor to absent

847. In hemolytic uremic syndrome all of the following are characteristic EXCEPT
A. bloody diarrhea
B. long-term sequelae are most often associated with the common neurologic manifestations
C. recurrent episodes are rare
D. hematuria
E. thrombocytopenia

848. Thrombocytosis is associated with all of the following EXCEPT
A. hereditary hemorrhagic telangiectasia
B. iron deficiency anemia
C. vitamin deficiency
D. megaloblastic anemia
E. platelet survival is usually normal

849. A disorder of platelet function should be suspected in the presence of all of the following EXCEPT
  A. bleeding time inappropriately prolonged for the platelet count
  B. a history of petechiae or ecchymosis
  C. poor clot retraction
  D. normal hemostatic screening tests
  E. epistaxis of moderate severity

850. Von Willebrand's disease (pseudohemophilia) is characterized by all of the following EXCEPT
  A. autosomal dominant inheritance
  B. bleeding diathesis is usually manifested by hemarthrosis
  C. reduction in plasma factor VIII
  D. deficient platelet adhesion
  E. menorrhagia may be a serious problem

851. Classic hemophilia (AHF deficiency, factor VIII deficiency) is usually associated with all of the following EXCEPT
  A. major joint hemarthroses are common
  B. abnormal partial thromboplastin time
  C. normal level of factor VIII antigen
  D. abnormal clotting time
  E. hematuria is a frequent manifestation

852. Christmas disease (PTC deficiency, factor IX deficiency) is associated with all of the following EXCEPT
  A. sex-linked transmission
  B. prolonged PTT
  C. the defect is corrected with stored plasma
  D. bleeding diathesis usually characterized by minor hemorrhages
  E. carriers may have level of PTC of 20% to 40% of normal

853. Factor XI deficiency (PTA deficiency) is associated with all of the following EXCEPT
  A. autosomal recessive inheritance
  B. it is the least common form of hemophilia
  C. the defect is connected with stored plasma
  D. hemorrhage problems are similar to those present in factor VIII or IX deficiencies, but symptoms are usually milder
  E. carriers rarely develop clinical bleeding

854. All the following statements are true regarding factor XII deficiency (Hageman trait) EXCEPT
   A. the bleeding problem is similar to factor XI deficiency
   B. abnormal PTT
   C. abnormal clotting time
   D. abnormal prothrombin consumption test
   E. patients are not subject to abnormal bleeding

855. Disseminated intravascular coagulation (DIC) may be associated with all of the following EXCEPT
   A. sickle cell anemia
   B. malignancy
   C. thrombocytopenia
   D. normal thrombin time (TT)
   E. polycythemic state

856. Which of the following is the first coagulation factor abnormality seen in liver disease?
   A. Factor VIII
   B. Factor VII
   C. Factor IX
   D. Fibrinogen
   E. Factor IX

DIRECTIONS: Each set of lettered headings below is followed by a list of numbered words or phrases. For each numbered word or phrase select

   A if the item is associated with (A) *only*,
   B if the item is associated with (B) *only*,
   C if the item is associated with *both* (A) *and* (B),
   D if the item is associated with *neither* (A) *nor* (B).

   A. Iron deficiency anemia
   B. Megaloblastic anemia
   C. Both
   D. Neither

857. Microcytic erythrocytes

858. Macrocytic erythrocytes

859. Commonly seen in premature infants

860. Treatment of the condition consists of dietary alteration alone

861. Associated with hypersegmented neutrophil nuclei

    A. Sickle cell disease
    B. Thalassemia
    C. Both
    D. Neither

862. An abnormality of the erythrocyte membrane

863. Patients have high incidence of pneumococcal and salmonella infections

864. Autosomal dominant mode of inheritance

865. Under normal circumstances heterozygotes have no symptoms

866. An abnormality of the structure of the beta-hemoglobin chain

    A. Hemophilia A (classic hemophilia)
    B. Von Willebrand's disease
    C. Both
    D. Neither

867. Decreased factor VIII activity

868. X-linked recessive mode of inheritance

869. Associated with thrombocytopenia

870. Autosomal dominant mode of inheritance

871. Prolonged prothrombin time

XVI: Blood and Blood-Forming Tissues Answers and Comments

787. B. RBC maturation reaches its peak in the liver at five months and begins in the marrow near the fifth month. *(REF. 1 — p. 1109)*

788. C. This humoral substance is produced primarily in the kidney. *(REF. 1 — p. 1110)*

789. A. Hemoglobin A is alpha 2 beta 2; hemoglobin A2 is alpha 2 delta 2; hemoglobin Gower 2 is alpha 2 epsilon 2; and hemoglobin Gower 1 contains four epsilon chains. *(REF. 1 — p. 1113)*

790. D. The average volume is 75 to 77 ml/kg. *(REF. 1 — p. 1112)*

791. D. There is a shift after birth owing to the decreased production of hemoglobin F, which has a lower affinity for 2, 3 diphosphoglycerate (important in modulating the interaction between hemoglobin and oxygen). In the other three conditions mentioned, the shift results from an increase in RBC concentration of 2, 3 DPG. *(REF. 1 — p. 1114)*

792. A. All the others are associated with a high MCV. *(REF. 1 — p. 1115)*

793. C. All others are usually associated with normal MCV and a low reticulocyte index. *(REF. 1 — p. 1116)*

794. D. An increase in serum unconjugated bilirubin is associated with extravascular hemolysis. *(REF. 1 — p. 1118)*

795. B. Benzidine and orthotoluidine reactions are excessively sensitive and may be positive in the absence of blood loss. *(REF. 1 — p. 1118)*

796. A. Vitamin E deficiency is characterized primarily by red cell destruction in the peripheral blood. Hemolysis occurs when there is insufficient vitamin E to protect the red cell membrane from oxidative injury. *(REF. 1 — p. 1119)*

797. E. Absorption is decreased by formation of insoluble phosphates and oxalates, which is favored by the alkaline environment of the small intestine. *(REF. 1 — p. 1119)*

798. A. In addition to a substantial diurnal variation, there is a marked day-to-day variability in the concentration of serum iron. The value would also be affected by a recent iron-rich meal. *(REF. 1 — p. 1122)*

799. C. A low concentration has been found only in association with iron deficiency. *(REF. 1 — p. 1123)*

800. C. Hypersegmentation of neutrophils is easy to detect on peripheral blood smear. Even when deficiencies of both iron and folate coexist, hypersegmentation is usually present, whereas red cell indices and serum folate levels become less reliable. *(REF. 1 — p. 1125)*

801. D. There is no clear inheritance pattern although endocrinopathies, and immune deficiencies may be present in siblings. *(REF. 1 — p. 1127)*

802. C. The gastric mucosa is normal with respect to morphology and secretory function. *(REF. 1 — p. 1127)*

803. A. Depression of serum vitamin B_{12} and the appearance of hypersegmented neutrophils are the earliest clinical manifestations. *(REF. 1 — p. 1127)*

804. D. Anemia is not consistently found, and when present it is mild and hypochromic. *(REF. 1 — p. 1129)*

805. C. The bone marrow stained for iron shows reduced or absent iron in erythroid precursors, despite the presence of RE iron. *(REF. 1 — p. 1130)*

806. A. Hepatomegaly is rare, adenopathy is absent, and splenomegaly is found in only 10% of cases. *(REF. 1 — p. 1130)*

807. D. Only about one in ten patients will develop acute leukemia. *(REF. 1 — p. 1132)*

808. C. The unknown maturational factor thought to be lacking in

272 / Blood and Blood-Forming Tissues

this disorder is probably not erythropoietin, since serum erythropoietin levels are unusually high, and the hormone has normal biologic activity in vivo. *(REF. 1 — p. 1132)*

809. A. Onset of acquired hypoplastic anemia is between the ages of four months and four years. *(REF. 1 — p. 1133)*

810. B. Of the five identified antigens C, D, E, e, c, the D antigen is the most antigenic and the one most often associated with disease. *(REF. 1 — p. 1135)*

811. C. Routine Rh testing generally fails to detect the D^u antigen because it is a weaker form of the D antigen and does not react with routine testing sera. The presence of D^u antigen means the mother is actually Rh-positive. *(REF. 1 — p. 1136)*

812. C. Islet cell hyperplasia and hyperinsulinism are present. It has been suggested that free hemoglobin in plasma binds to and inactivates insulin; the compensatory increase in insulin production causes islet cell hyperplasia. *(REF. 1 — p. 1137)*

813. B. Although reticulocytopenia may be observed during the initial stages, the reticulocyte count is usually elevated. Platelets may be decreased, and total leukocyte counts may be either increased or decreased. *(REF. 1 — p. 1146)*

814. C. Cephalothin usually results in a positive Coombs' test by the nonimmunologic adsorption of proteins on the surface of the red cell. This is not associated with hemolysis, and only in rare situations does it act as a hapten with resulting hemolysis. *(REF. 1 — p. 1147)*

815. B. Leukopenia and thrombocytopenia are commonly seen. *(REF. 1 — p. 1148)*

816. D. Hypertonicity of plasma increases intracellular concentration of hemoglobin S, and hypertonic dehydration promotes sickling. *(REF. 1 — p. 1149)*

817. D. Salmonella osteomyelitis rarely progresses to sepsis. *(REF. 1 — p. 1151)*

818. A. Pneumococci is most likely a result of failure of the spleen to produce opsonizing antibodies. *(REF. 1 — p. 1151)*

819. C. The hemoglobin, hematocrit — red cell indices — and reticulocyte count are normal in sickle cell trait. *(REF. 1 — p. 1154)*

820. B. Life expectancy is normal. *(REF. 1 — p. 1156)*

821. C. The relative percentage of A2 hemoglobin may be reduced, normal, or elevated; therefore, it is of little diagnostic value. *(REF. 1 — p. 1156)*

822. D. The MCV is at or below the lower limit of normal for age and the MCHC is greater than normal and often as high as 37% to 38%. *(REF. 1 — p. 1164)*

823. A. Osmotic fragility of fresh erythrocytes is normal but is increased after incubation at 37°C. *(REF. 1 — p. 1165)*

824. C. Red cell morphology is characterized by the presence of acanthocytes; however, they are also relatively common and reversible findings in infants with an adequate supply of vitamin E and are therefore of limited help in diagnosis. *(REF. 1 — p. 1167)*

825. B. Between hemolytic episodes, anemia is absent, and RBC survival may be normal. *(REF. 1 — p. 1169)*

826. B. Newborns are more susceptible because hemoglobin F is more readily oxidized than hemoglobin A. *(REF. 1 — p. 1175)*

827. B. Antibodies of the IgG class as well as C3 are the most important opsonins. *(REF. 1 — p. 1176)*

828. C. Eosinophilia usually appears to reflect some type of hypersensitivity reaction. Eosinophils do ingest antigen-antibody complexes. *(REF. 1 — p. 1177)*

829. A. Pulmonary infections and an abnormal sweat test are not characteristic. *(REF. 1 — p. 1180)*

830. C. Despite their morphologic abnormalities, neutrophils retain their ability to phagocytose and kill bacteria. *(REF. 1 — p. 1181)*

831. C. At present, the combination of staphylococci and BHS are more common. *(REF. 1 — p. 1182)*

832. D. The response to chemotherapy is not as good as in the adult variety, and the median survival time is less than that for the adult. *(REF. 1 — p. 1183)*

833. C. Sixty percent of the cases occur initially in the neck, with axillary and inguinal adenopathies less frequent. *(REF. 1 — p. 1191)*

834. D. As in Hodgkin's, the male-to-female ratio is 3:1. *(REF. 1 — p. 1193)*

835. A. Diffuse bone marrow infiltration develops in about one third of children and is especially common in those who initially have primary tumors in the mediastinum. *(REF. 1 — p. 1194)*

836. D. Thirty percent of normal newborns and 15% of infants below six months of age will have palpable spleens. *(REF. 1 — p. 1195)*

837. B. Pneumococci are responsible for over half of the cases of sepsis in asplenia. *(REF. 1 — p. 1196)*

838. A. Von Willebrand's disease is inherited as an autosomal dominant trait. Factor VIII and IX deficiencies are sex-linked disorders; factors V and VII are autosomal recessive disorders. *(REF. 1 — p. 1200)*

839. E. PT measures thrombin generation in the extrinsic pathway. Factor IX is part of the intrinsic clotting system. *(REF. 1 — p. 1201)*

840. B. PTT measures thrombin generation in the intrinsic pathway and is a function of all the coagulation factors except factor VII. *(REF. 1 — p. 1201)*

841. A. Vitamin K-dependent factor includes factors II, VII, IX, X, which are low at birth and often fall to even lower levels during the first week, unless vitamin K is given soon after birth. *(REF. 1 — p. 1201)*

842. B. PTT may be abnormal owing to variable deficiency of factor VIII. *(REF. 1 — p. 1201)*

843. B. Single or multiple joint swelling is present but is a result of periarticular involvement rather than intra-articular bleeding. Joints may be puffy, warm, painful, and tender. *(REF. 1 — p. 1204)*

844. A. Platelets are normal. The generalized vascular disorder results from acute aseptic vasculitis involving arterioles and capillaries. *(REF. 1 — p. 1204)*

845. D. Enlargement of spleen and lymph nodes is rare. *(REF. 1 — p. 1205)*

846. D. Bone marrow exam may reveal an increased number of megakaryocytes with a predominance of immature forms. *(REF. 1 — p. 1206)*

847. B. Long-term sequelae are restricted to chronic renal disease. *(REF. 1 — p. 1207)*

848. A. In hereditary hemorrhagic telangiectasia, the platelet count is normal, but there is decreased platelet aggregation. *(REF. 1 — p. 1209)*

849. D. Screening tests are usually normal except for bleeding time, which may be prolonged. *(REF. 1 — p. 1208)*

850. B. Nosebleeds and easy bruising are the most common manifestations; hemarthroses are rare. *(REF. 1 — p. 1209)*

851. D. Whole blood clotting time is markedly prolonged only in severe hemophilia; only 1% to 2% of normal factor VIII levels will produce a normal clotting time. *(REF. 1 — p. 1210)*

852. D. Clinical manifestations are indistinguishable for classic hemophilia, i.e., major hemorrhages in joints. *(REF. 1 — p. 1212)*

853. C. Treatment is with fresh frozen plasma and deficiency is not connected with stored plasma. *(REF. 1 — p. 1212)*

854. A. Patients are not subject to abnormal bleeding. The problem is usually found in screening tests for bleeding difficulties. *(REF. 1 — p. 1212)*

855. D. TT estimates the amount and function of fibrinogen and is particularly sensitive to the presence of fibrin degradation products, which are elevated in DIC. *(REF. 1 — p. 1214)*

856. B. Factor VII has a biologic half-life of four hours, and its

276 / Blood and Blood-Forming Tissues

deficiency is manifested by a prolonged prothrombin time. *(REF. 1 — p. 1213)*

857. A. Megaloblastic anemia is associated with macrocytic
858. B. erythrocytes and hypersegmented neutrophil nuclei. Iron
859. C. deficiency anemia is associated with microcytic erythro-
860. D. cytes. Both conditions are commonly seen in premature in-
861. B. fants, and neither should be treated with dietary therapy
         alone once anemia is present. *(REF. 1 — p. 1119)*

862. D. Both sickle cell disease and thalassemia are abnormalities
863. A. of hemoglobin synthesis, and both are inherited as auto-
864. D. somal recessive traits. Sickle cell patients have a high in-
865. A. cidence of pneumococcal and salmonella infections, and
866. A. the heterozygotes are asymptomatic. Sickle cell has abnor-
         malities of beta-chain synthesis only and they do not in-
volve the RBC membrane. *(REF. 1 — pp. 1149, 1151, 1155, 1156)*

867. C. Hemophilia A has an X-linked mode of inheritance and
868. A. decreased factor VIII activity. Von Willebrand's disease is
869. D. autosomal dominant and also has decreased factor VIII
870. B. activity. Neither is associated with thrombocytopenia or
871. D. prolonged prothrombin times. *(REF. 1 — p. 1209)*

XVII: Kidney and Urinary Tract

DIRECTIONS: Each of the questions or incomplete statements below is followed by five suggested answers or completions. Select the **one** that is **BEST** in each case.

872. Which of the following variables is the major determinant of the glomerular filtration rate (GFR)?
    A. Permeability of the glomerular basement membrane
    B. Intracapillary hydrostatic pressure
    C. Intracapsular hydrostatic pressure
    D. Colloid osmotic pressure
    E. Serum osmolarity

873. Which of the following solutes is generally considered best for accurate determination of GFR?
    A. Inulin
    B. Mannitol
    C. Creatinine
    D. Creatine phosphate
    E. Cyanocobalamin

874. Urinary excretion of potassium is increased under all the following conditions EXCEPT
    A. persistent increased intake of potassium
    B. increased amounts of circulatory mineralocorticoid hormones
    C. metabolic acidosis
    D. administration of diuretics such as hydrochlorothiazide
    E. respiratory alkalosis

875. Which of the following is NOT associated with plasma hyper-osmolality?
   A. Vasopressin release by posterior pituitary gland
   B. Swelling of osmoreceptor cells in the hypothalamus
   C. Production of concentrated urine of decreased volume
   D. Increase amount of solute-free water to plasma
   E. Decrease of the intracellular fluid volume

876. The major influence of vasopressin on water balance occurs at which of the following points?
   A. Glomular basement membrane
   B. Proximal convoluted renal tubule
   C. Descending loop of Henle
   D. Ascending loop of Henle
   E. Distal convoluted tubule

877. Factors that cause an increase in the rate of H^+ secretion by the proximal tubule and lead to increased HCO_3^- reabsorption with consequent elevation of plasma HCO_3^- include all of the following EXCEPT
   A. hypokalemia
   B. inhibition of carbonic anhydrase
   C. metabolic acidosis
   D. reduction in effective arterial blood volume (i.e., after hemorrhage with burns)
   E. administration of mineralocorticoids

878. Proteinuria is usually greatest in which of the following conditions?
   A. Pyelonephritis
   B. Polycystic kidney
   C. Acute poststreptococcal glomerulonephritis
   D. Nephrolithiasis
   E. Early urate nephropathy

879. Orthostatic (postural) proteinuria is characterized by all of the following EXCEPT
   A. the usual age of detection is in the second decade of life
   B. it is usually a subtle manifestation of chronic renal disease
   C. there is an increased amount of urinary protein when patient is in upright position
   D. proteinuria is resolved when the patient is in a recumbent position
   E. total 24-hour urinary excretion of protein seldom exceeds 1,000 mg

880. Which of the following statements regarding hematuria is NOT true?
   A. If casts are present the source of hematuria must be the kidney
   B. Bright red urine with clots usually suggests renal or upper urinary tract source of bleeding
   C. The additional finding of proteinuria usually suggests a renal source
   D. The most common neoplasm associated with hematuria is Wilms' tumor
   E. It can be a cause of anemia

881. Which of the following immunoglobulins may be fixed by complement in the glomerulus?
   A. IgA
   B. IgG
   C. IgE
   D. IgD
   E. None of the above

882. Which of the following findings is considered the essential common feature shared by all manifestations of the nephrotic syndrome?
   A. Marked proteinuria
   B. Hyperlipidemia
   C. Hypertension
   D. Hypoproteinuria
   E. Edema

883. Which of the following proteins is LEAST readily excreted in the nephrotic syndrome?
   A. Albumin
   B. IgG
   C. Lipoprotein
   D. Transferrin
   E. IgE

884. Of the cardinal features of the nephrotic syndrome, which of the following is considered the most variable during the course of the disease?
   A. Proteinuria
   B. Edema
   C. Hyperlipemia
   D. Hypoproteinemia
   E. Increased renin excretion

885. All of the following are consistent with the diagnosis of idiopathic nephrotic syndrome of childhood EXCEPT
   A. onset is between two and eight years of age
   B. pathologic renal changes are minimal by light microscopy
   C. depression of B'C globulin
   D. hypertension is unusual
   E. hyperlipidemia

886. Membranoproliferative glomerulonephritis is characterized by all of the following EXCEPT
   A. pathologic thickening of the glomerular basement membrane
   B. hypertension is common
   C. serum complement level is normal
   D. onset in late childhood
   E. nephrotic syndrome

887. Which of the following M-serotypes of streptococci is most frequently associated with postpyoderma acute glomerulonephritis?
   A. 12
   B. 4
   C. 25
   D. 3
   E. 49

888. Of the following antistreptococcal enzymes, which is most often elevated in acute nephritis induced by skin infection (as opposed to pharyngeal infection)?
    A. Anti-deoxyribonuclease B (DNase-B)
    B. Anti-streptolysin-O (ASO)
    C. Anti-nicotinamide-adenine dinucleotidase (NADase)
    D. Anti-hyaluronidase
    E. Anti-diphosphopyridine nucleotidase (DPNase)

889. Acute poststreptococcal glomerulonephritis is characterized by all of the following EXCEPT
    A. specific streptococcal antigens are found at the site of IgG and BC globulin deposits in glomerulus
    B. marked depression of C3 and terminal components of complement
    C. usually a beginning resolution of abnormal glomerular changes within two to three weeks of clinical onset of disease
    D. ESR is usually elevated
    E. red blood cell casts in the urine

890. The nephritis of anaphylactoid purpura is manifested by all of the following EXCEPT
    A. severity of the nephritis correlates well with the amount of protein excreted
    B. serum BC globulin level is depressed
    C. prognosis is good owing to self-limiting character of the nephritis
    D. nephritis occurs in about 50% of children with anaphylactoid purpura
    E. gross or microscopic hematuria

891. The pathophysiology of the hemolytic-uremic syndrome is associated with all of the following EXCEPT
    A. immune mechanisms are considered important in the pathogenesis
    B. hemolytic anemia is Coombs-negative
    C. thrombocytopenia probably results from platelet aggregation within damaged vessels
    D. renal microangiopathy affecting small arterioles and glomerular capillaries is the most consistent pathologic change
    E. uncertain pathogenesis

892. Which the following laboratory tests is normal in hemolytic-uremic syndrome?
  A. Platelet count
  ✓ B. BC
  C. BUN
  D. Serum creatinine
  E. Serum lipid concentration

893. Renal tubular acidosis (RTA) may be accurately described by and associated with all of the following EXCEPT
  A. a clinical syndrome of sustained hyperchloremic metabolic acidosis in the absence of significant reduction in glomerular filtration rate
  B. distal and proximal RTA occur either as primary abnormalities in urine acidification or as secondary disorders to systemic disease or intoxication
  ✓ C. distal RTA, compared to proximal RTA, is more commonly secondary to a systemic disorder or toxin
  D. nephrocalcinosis is seen in distal RTA
  E. failure to thrive

894. Which of the following laboratory findings is NOT associated with distal renal tubular acidosis?
  A. Urine pH of 6.0 or higher
  B. Aminoaciduria
  C. Hypokalemia
  D. Hypocalcemia
  E. Hypocapnia

895. The Fanconi syndrome, due to a complex proximal tubular dysfunction, is associated with all of the following EXCEPT
  A. renal tubular acidosis with bicarbonaturia
  B. glycosuria with hyperglycemia
  C. phosphaturia with hypophosphatemia
  D. generalized aminoaciduria without elevated plasma levels of amino acids
  E. hypouricemia

896. Nephrogenic diabetes insipidus is associated with all of the following EXCEPT
  A. unresponsiveness of proximal tubule to vasopressin
  B. decreased production of cyclic 3,5-AMP, which mediates the permeability of distal tubule to the passive diffusion of luminal water into medullary interstitium
  C. normal transport of tubular sodium and chloride
  D. no consistent renal pathologic changes are demonstrated
  E. hypernatremia

897. Renal glycosuria (renal glucosuria) may be characterized by all of the following EXCEPT
  A. hereditary defect in tubular glucose transport
  B. glucose tolerance curve is either normal or flat
  C. urinary loss of glucose has little effect on blood glucose concentration
  D. all urine specimens contain glucose regardless of normal blood glucose concentrations
  E. inherited usually as sex-linked

898. The autosomal recessive defect in amino acid transport associated with cystinuria is characterized by all of the following EXCEPT
  A. amino acids involved include cystine, lysine, arginine, ornithine and cystine-homocysteine mixed disulfide
  B. a positive urine cyanide-nitroprusside test is pathognomonic
  C. usual presentation is that of ureteral colic or obstruction
  D. both sexes are affected
  E. gastrointestinal amino acid transport is also affected

899. Which of the following is NOT associated with Alport's syndrome?
  A. Most common of the heritable renal diseases
  B. High-frequency sensorineural deafness
  C. Cataracts
  D. Wide geographic distributions are found in patients of different racial and ethnic backgrounds
  E. Onset during second decade

900. Childhood polycystic kidney disease is characterized by all of the following EXCEPT

    A. liver involvement is common and is associated with dilatation of portal bile ducts

    B. renal disease presenting at adolescence or later is relatively milder than that in infants

    C. it is an autosomal recessive disorder

    D. associated lower urinary system abnormalities are common

    E. hematuria may be present

901. Acute pyelonephritis in children is associated with all of the following EXCEPT

    A. impaired migration of polymorphonuclear leukocytes and phagocytosis because of medullary hypertonicity

    B. it is often secondary to reflux from lower urinary tract

    C. impaired ability to concentrate urine

    D. it is rarely associated with meatal stenosis

    E. abdominal pain

902. Renal vein thrombosis in infants is characterized by all of the following EXCEPT

    A. it is probably related to venous stasis secondary to shock, septicemia, or dehydration

    B. edema and hypertension

    C. thrombocytopenia

    D. disseminated intravascular coagulopathy

    E. an enlarged kidney that does not visualize on intravenous urography

---

DIRECTIONS: Each group of questions below consists of five lettered headings followed by a list of numbered words, phrases or statements. For **each** numbered word, phrase, or statement, select the **one** lettered heading that is most closely associated with it. Each lettered heading may be selected once, more than once, or not at all.

    A. Goodpasture's syndrome
    B. Hemolytic-uremic syndrome
    C. Systemic lupus erythematosus
    D. Acute poststreptococcal glomerulonephritis
    E. Polyarteritis nodosa

903. Majority of patients have no permanent impairment of renal function

904. Associated with nephritis and pulmonary hemorrhage

905. The female/male ratio for this type of nephritis is 4:1

906. Thought to be a hypersensitivity reaction involving medium-sized vessels in its chronic form

907. Usually preceded by a gastroenteritis prodrome

908. Steroids and cytotoxic immunosuppressant drugs are now recommended as therapy

    A. Recurrent hematuria
    B. Hyperuricemia nephropathy
    C. Sickle cell disease
    D. Hepatorenal syndrome
    E. Potassium nephropathy

909. Presumed anoxic injury causes the concentrating defect observed in patients with this condition

910. This reversible condition affecting mainly the proximal convuluted tubule can be caused by hyperadrenalism

911. Associated with cancer chemotherapy and Lesch-Nyhan syndrome

912. Believed to be caused by glomerular immunoglobulin deposition

913. Patients unusually prone to develop pyelonephritis

914. Although rare in childhood, it is thought to be caused by decreased renal blood flow

    A. Hydrocele
    B. Posterior urethral valves
    C. Horseshoe kidney
    D. Prune-belly syndrome
    E. Vesicourethral reflux

915. Absence of the abdominal wall musculature, bilateral un-descended testes, and urinary tract anomalies

916. Found in high frequency in patients with Turner's syndrome

917. Spontaneous cure is likely and usually occurs in the first year of life

918. Provides a ready pathway for ascending urinary tract infections

919. A congenital abnormality of the verumontanum

920. Transillumination can be diagnostic

XVII: Kidney and Urinary Tract
Answers and Comments

872. B. Intracapillary hydrostatic pressure is the major determinant of GFR and is dependent on the systemic aortic blood pressure and on the afferent and efferent arteriolar tone. *(REF. 3 — p. 1170)*

873. A. Inulin, a fructose polymer with a mean molecular weight of 5,000 is completely filtrable, as are smaller molecules. The concentration of these substances is virtually the same in the ultrafiltrates as in the plasma. *(REF. 2 — p. 1478)*

874. C. Potassium excretion is reduced during respiratory and metabolic acidosis. During alkalosis hydrogen is exchanged for potassium; therefore, the amount of potassium available for secretion increases, and excretion is enhanced. *(REF. 2 — p. 1485)*

875. B. Osmoreceptor cells of hypothalamus shrink when the effective osmotic pressure of the plasma is elevated. *(REF. 3 — p. 1173)*

876. E. The major influence of vasopressin on water balance occurs in the distal convoluted tubule where, in a state of antidiuresis, approximately 15% of filtered water is reabsorbed as the luminal urine becomes isosmotic. *(REF. 3 — p. 1174)*

877. B. Inhibition of carbonic anhydrase is associated with H^+ secretion and decreased reabsorption of HCO_3^-. *(REF. 3 — p. 1175)*

878. C. In all the other choices presented, proteinuria may be absent or usually mild. *(REF. 2 — p. 1482)*

879. B. May be normal variant and most children are healthy and have no underlying renal pathology. *(REF. 2 — p. 1483)*

880. B. Bright red urine, with or without clots, suggests an extrarenal source of bleeding. *(REF. 2 — pp. 1483–1484)*

881. B. IgG and IgM may be fixed by complement in the glomerulus. *(REF. 2 — p. 1491)*

882. A. Proteinuria usually to the extent of 2 gm/m^2/24 hrs or more. *(REF. 2 — p. 1494)*

883. C. Generally, plasma proteins of low molecular weights are excreted more readily. Lipoproteins are considered to be of high molecular weight. *(REF. 2 — p. 1494)*

884. B. Although edema dominates the clinical picture from a layman's point of view it should be regarded as a secondary manifestation the presence or absence of which is influenced by several factors. *(REF. 2 — p. 1494)*

885. C. Serum level of BC globulin is usually normal. Additionally, immunopathologic studies reveal an absence of deposits of immune globulins or complement components. *(REF. 2 — pp. 1495–1496)*

886. C. Depression of complement includes C3, C5 and C9. Immunopathologic studies show granular deposition of BC globulin in proliferating mesangial region. *(REF. 2 — pp. 1499–1500)*

887. E. The lower numbered M-serotypes are generally the pharyngeal strains associated with acute nephritis. *(REF. 2 — p. 1502)*

888. A. ASO and anti-NADase responses are irregular or weak following impetigo. There is usually a good anti-hyaluronidase response following skin infections also. The response to DPNase is usually better following pharyngeal infections with streptococci. *(REF. 2 — p. 1503)*

889. A. Specific streptococcal antigens are not found at the site of IgG and BC deposition. *(REF. 2 — p. 1503)*

890. B. Serum B, C level is normal. Glomerular deposits of IgG and BC have been seen but do not have characteristic location or appearance seen in other forms of immune complex injury. *(REF. 2 — p. 1511)*

891. A. Immune mechanisms are not considered operative, since there is no deposition of complement components or immunoglobulins at the site of the arteriolar or glomerular lesions. *(REF. 2 — pp. 1512–1513)*

892. B. Serum BC is usually normal, although there may be a decrease in total hemolytic complement. *(REF. 2 — pp. 1513–1514)*

893. C. Proximal RTA also occurs as a primary isolated defect, but is more commonly secondary to a systemic disorder or toxin. It is usually associated with other features of impaired proximal tubular transport. *(REF. 2 — pp. 1515–1516)*

894. B. Fanconi syndrome may be associated with *proximal* RTA and therefore may include aminoaciduria, glucosuria, phosphaturia, tubular proteinuria, and hypophosphatemia. These are not usually seen in distal RTA. *(REF. 2 — p. 1517)*

895. B. Glycosuria occurs without hyperglycemia. *(REF. 2 — p. 1519)*

896. A. Primary defect is believed to be an enzymatic or biochemical abnormality in *distal* tubular function. *(REF. 2 — pp. 1519–1520)*

897. E. In some families the condition is inherited as an autosomal dominant, in others an autosomal recessive mode is probable. *(REF. 2 — p. 1521)*

898. B. This test is also positive in homocystinuria and acetonuria. *(REF. 2 — p. 1522)*

899. E. The mean age of onset is six years, but it has been noted as early as five months. *(REF. 2 — p. 1523)*

900. D. The renal pelves, ureters, bladder and urethra are normal. *(REF. 2 — p. 1530)*

901. C. Decreased concentrating ability is usually associated with chronic pyelonephritis and is most likely a result of damage to the renal medulla, progressive interstitial scarring, and nephron destruction. *(REF. 2 — p. 1546)*

902. B. Edema and hypertension are usually absent. *(REF. 2 — pp. 1553–1554)*

903. D. The ratio of females to males with SLE is 4:1. It is now
904. A. recommended that SLE patients with renal involvement be
905. C. treated with steroids, and if no response is observed
906. E. cytotoxic immunosuppressants are used. Goodpasture's
907. B. syndrome is associated with nephritis and pulmonary hem-

908. C. orrhage. In the hemolytic-uremic syndrome there is usually a prodrome of gastroenteritis. The pathology of chronic
polyarteritis nodosa involves a hypersensitivity reaction of the
medium-sized vessel. The majority of patients with acute poststreptococcal glomerulonephritis recover without permanent renal
damage. The other listed conditions are associated with permanent
renal impairment. *(REE. 1 — p. 1263)*

909. C. Patients with hyperuremic nephropathy are especially
910. E. prone to develop pyelonephritis. This condition is seen
911. B. commonly in cancer patients receiving cytolytic drugs and
912. A. in patients with Lesch-Nyhan syndrome. Nephropathy
913. B. seen in sickle cell disease is believed to be caused by hypox-
914. D. ic injury and results in a concentrating defect early on. The
hepatorenal syndrome, although rare in childhood is
thought to be caused by decreased renal blood flow. Potassium
nephropathy affects the epithelium of the proximal tubule and may
be seen in hyperadrenalism. The condition is reversible. Biopsies of
patients with recurrent hematuria have been shown to be laden with
glomerular immunoglobulin deposits. *(REF. 1 — p. 1238)*

915. D. Hydroceles can be diagnosed by physical examination and
916. C. transillumination and carry a high spontaneous cure rate
917. A. during the first year of life. The prune-belly triad consists
918. E. of absence of the abdominal musculature, undescended
919. B. testes, and various renal anomalies. Visicoureteral reflux
920. A. provides a ready pathway for bacteria in ascending urinary
tract infection. Posterior urethral values are a congenital
malformation of the verumontanum. Horseshoe kidneys are found
with high frequency in patients with the Turner's syndrome. *(REF. 1
— pp. 1339–1346)*

XVIII: Bones and Joints

DIRECTIONS: Each of the questions or incomplete statements below is followed by five suggested answers or completions. Select the one that is BEST in each case.

921. Components of congenital clubfoot include all of the following EXCEPT
    A. metarsus adductus
    B. calcaneovalgus
    C. plantar flexion
    D. equinovarus deformity of ankle
    E. relative rigidity of position

922. The most common organism associated with osteomyelitis in children is
    A. *S. aureus*
    B. Group A beta-hemolytic streptococcus
    C. salmonella
    D. *H. influenzae*
    E. *Streptococcus viridans*

923. Chondroectodermal dysplasia (Ellis-van Creveld syndrome) differs from achondroplasia in all of the following EXCEPT
    A. the presence of congenital heart disease
    B. short stature
    C. normal skull growth and configuration
    D. polydactyly
    E. hypoplasia of the nails, teeth, and hair

924. Which of the following conditions is associated with normal platelet function?
A. Thrombocytosis
B. Vitamin C deficiency
C. Abnormal globulins, i.e., macroglobulinemia
D. Disseminated intravascular coagulopathy
E. Von Willebrand's disease

925. All of the following are characteristic of cleidocranial dysplasia EXCEPT
A. Poorly formed dentition
B. widely spaced eyes
C. failure of development of clavicle
D. soft calvarium
E. mental retardation

926. Marfan's syndrome and homocystinuria share all of the following clinical features EXCEPT
A. mental retardation
B. ectopic lenses
C. aortic aneurysm
D. excessive length of tubular bones
E. genetic transmission to offspring

927. Hypophosphatasia resembles rickets in all of the following EXCEPT
A. low alkaline phosphatase
B. rachitic rosary
C. short stature
D. enlargement of joints
E. bowleg

928. Coxa plana (Legg-Calvé-Perthes disease) is characterized by all of the following EXCEPT
A. limitation of abduction and of external rotation of hip
B. it rarely develops before three years
C. hip pain is frequently referred to medial side of ipsilateral knee
D. it is more frequent in boys than girls
E. bilateral hip involvement common

929. Köhler's disease represents osteochondrosis of which of the following bones?
   A. Tuberosity of tibia
   B. Tarsal navicular
   C. Patella
   D. Medial tibial condyle
   E. Metatarsal

930. Infantile cortical hyperostosis is characterized by all of the following EXCEPT
   A. high erythrocyte sedimentation rate
   B. increased alkaline phosphatase
   C. lymphadenopathy
   D. external thickening of bony cortex
   E. negative bacterial, viral, and serologic studies

931. Which of the following organisms is associated most often in acute pyarthrosis in children under two years?
   A. *S. aureus*
   B. Beta-hemolytic streptococci
   C. Pneumococci
   D. *H. influenzae*
   E. *S. viridans*

DIRECTIONS: Each group of questions below consists of five lettered headings followed by a list of numbered words, phrases or statements. For **each** numbered word, phrase or statement, select the **one** lettered heading that is most closely associated with it. Each lettered heading may be selected once, more than once, or not at all.

   A. Scaphocephaly
   B. Acrocephalosyndactyly
   C. Crouzon's disease
   D. Lacunar skull
   E. Platybasia

932. Meningocele is the most commonly associated defect

933. Early fusion of the sagittal suture only

934. Autosomal dominant disorder involving the maxilla, cranial bones, and lips

935. Assimilation of atlas into occiput

936. Pointing of the head and abnormalities of the sutures, hands, and feet

937. Associated with brainstem encroachment

    A. Achondroplasia
    B. Spondyloepiphyseal dysplasia
    C. Chondroectodermal dysplasia
    D. Chondrodystrophia calcificans congenita
    E. Asphyxiating thoracic dystrophy

938. Syndrome includes polydactyly and congenital heart disease

939. Carpals and tarsals replaced by small scattered calcified spots and short limbs

940. Disproportionate growth at the base of the skull results in a depressed nasal bridge and bulging forehead

941. Chondrodysplasia with very short ribs, polydactyly, and clefts in the acetalbulum and metaphyses of the long bones

942. Infant appears normal at birth

943. Recessively inherited chondrodysplasia often associated with cataracts

    A. Osgood-Schlatter disease
    B. Subluxation of the head of the radius
    C. Legg-Calvé-Perthes disease
    D. Slipped femoral epiphysis
    E. Congenital subluxation of the hip

944. Aseptic necrosis of the capital femoral epiphysis

945. Benign condition completely resolved after simple reduction

946. Believed to be caused by chronic trauma to the anterior tibial tubercle

947. Associated with the Ortolani's click

948. Occurs typically in the "overlarge" adolescent, with the insidious onset of knee pain

949. Disease of unknown cause occurring most frequently in males between the ages of four and ten years

XVIII: Bones and Joints
Answers and Comments

921. B. Calcaneovalgus refers to dorsiflexion with lateral deviation; the opposite is the case in clubfoot. *(REF. 1 — p. 1992)*

922. A. *S. aureus* accounts for 70% to 90% of cases in otherwise normal children. *REF. 1 — p. 1999)*

923. B. In both conditions there is shortening of extremities but in dysplasia the shortening occurs more prominently in the distal than in the proximal portions. *(REF. 1 — p. 2007)*

924. A. Platelet function is normal in thrombocytosis. *(REF. 1 — p. 1209)*

925. E. Intelligence is normal. Despite the softness of the calvarium, it rarely results in brain damage. Convulsive disorders and development of neurologic abnormalities occasionally occur. *(REF. 1 — p. 2013)*

926. A. Universal mental retardation and urinary excretion of homocystine are features of homocystinuria. In addition the latter is transmitted as an autosomal recessive trait as opposed to autosomal dominant in the former. *(REF. 1 — p. 2014)*

927. A. Alkaline phosphatase is normal in vitamin D-deficient as well as vitamin D-resistant rickets. Low levels of alkaline phosphatase are associated with defective transformation of cartilage and bone, premature shedding of deciduous teeth, and an abnormal metabolite in the urine. *(REF. 1 — p. 2015)*

928. E. Bilateral involvement occurs only in 10% of cases. *(REF. 1 — p. 2019)*

929. B. Osteochondrosis of the tibia is Osgood-Schlatter disease; osteochondrosis of the patella is Syndig-Larsen disease; pseudo-osteochondrosis of the medial tibial condyle is Blount's disease; and pseudo-osteochondrosis of a single vertebral body is Calvé's disease. *(REF. 1 — p. 2021)*

930. C. There is no lymphadenopathy in any phase of the disease. *(REF. 1 — p. 2022)*

931. D. Staphylococci are most often found in children over two years of age. *(REF. 1 — p. 2026)*

932. D. Platybasia involves assimilation of the atlas into the oc-
933. A. ciput and possible encroachment of the brainstem.
934. C. Scaphocephaly is caused by premature closure of the sagit-
935. E. tal suture. Crouzon's disease (craniofacial dysostosis) is a
936. B. deformity of the maxilla, acrocephaly, and short upper lip
937. E. and protruding lower lip. Acrocephalosyndactyly involves
pointing of the head, syndactyly of the hands and feet, and abnormalities of the sutures. Lacunar skull is most commonly associated with meningocele. *(REF. 2 — pp. 1828-1829)*

938. C. Chondrodystrophia calcificans congenita is a recessively
939. D. inherited chrondrodysplasia (associated with cataracts) in
940. A. which the tarsal and carpal bones are replaced by scattered
941. E. calcified spots. Short limbs are also part of the conditions.
942. B. In achondroplasia, an abnormal skull is formed by dyspro-
943. D. portionate growth at its base. Chondroectodermal dys-
plasia is associated with polydactyly, congenital heart disease, and defective dentition. Asphyxiating thoracic dystrophy (Jeune syndrome) is characterized by short ribs, short long bones, and cleft-like lesions in the acetabulum and metaphysis of long bones. In spondyloepiphyseal dysplasia, the infant appears normal at birth. *(REF. 2 — pp. 1832-1838)*

944. C. Legg-Calvé-Perthes disease is of unknown etiology and
945. D. most commonly affects males between four and ten years
946. A. of age. The lesion found is aseptic necrosis of the hip. Slip-
947. E. ped capital femoral epiphysis occurs with an insidious
948. D. onset of knee pain in the "overlarge" adolescent. Subluxa-
949. C. tion of the head of the radius is a benign condition.
Congenital subluxation of the hip is suggested by a click heard or felt while performing the Ortolani maneuver. Osgood-Schlatter disease is believed to be caused by chronic trauma to the antitibial tubercle. *(REF. 2 — pp. 1815-1819)*

XIX: Eye

DIRECTIONS: Each of the questions or incomplete statements below is followed by five suggested answers or completions. Select the one that is **BEST** in each case.

950. Visual acuity can probably be first estimated at age
    A. six to eight weeks
    B. four to five months
    C. six to nine months
    D. three to four years
    E. seven to eight years

951. Approximately what percentage of the adult-sized eye is the newborn eye?
    A. 25%
    B. 30%
    C. 50%
    D. 75%
    E. 95%

952. The normal child has a visual acuity approximating that of the adult (20/20) at age
    A. seven to eight weeks
    B. three to four months
    C. 18 to 24 months
    D. two to three years
    E. four to five years

953. All of the following are correct statements regarding color vision EXCEPT
   A. color vision deficits may lead to learning disturbances in school
   B. color blindness is usually partial
   C. color blindness is usually of the red-green deficiency type
   D. color blindness is no longer recognized as a sex-linked disorder
   E. there is no suitable treatment for color blindness

954. Leukokoria is associated with
   A. retinoblastoma
   B. interstitial keratitis
   C. ocular albinism
   D. conjunctivitis
   E. blepharitis

955. Defective closure of the optic fissure produces a
   A. anophthalmos
   B. cyclopia
   C. coloboma
   D. microphthalmos
   E. cataract

956. The most common anomaly of the eyelids is
   A. entropion
   B. congenital ptosis
   C. ectropion
   D. palpebral coloboma
   E. blepharophimosis

957. A child is seen with a very peculiar form of eyelid ptosis. When the mouth is opened or when the jaw is moved to the side opposite the ptosis, there is elevation of the ptotic lid. This is called the
   A. Marcus Gunn phenomenon
   B. trichiasis
   C. Waardenburg syndrome
   D. epicanthal phenomenon
   E. Horner's syndrome

958. The common stye is the
- A. angular blepharitis
- B. external hordeolum
- C. chalazion
- D. distichia
- E. ectropion

959. A child presents with scaling and inflammation of the muco-cutaneous borders of the angles of the lids. Microscopic examination of the scrapings reveals large gram-negative diplobacilli with no leukocytes. The most likely diagnosis is infection with
- A. *S. aureus*
- B. *Haemophilus duplex*
- C. *Pediculus pubis*
- D. *P. capitis*
- E. *N. gonorrhoeae*

960. Silver nitrate conjunctivitis
- A. requires immediate therapy with corticosteroids
- B. usually causes cataracts
- C. may result in perforation of the globe
- D. causes blindness in 50% of infants
- E. requires conservative therapy

961. All of the following are correct statements about trachoma EXCEPT
- A. it is the most common cause of impaired vision
- B. in some localities it is endemic
- C. it is caused by herpes simplex
- D. the acute phase is followed by a chronic low-grade inflammation
- E. corticosteroids are contraindicated

962. Blueness of the sclera indicates
- A. trisomy 18 syndrome
- B. vitamin C deficiency
- C. increased intraocular pressure
- D. hypercalcemia
- E. no specific pathology

963. The fundus of the normal newborn may reveal all of the following EXCEPT
   A. the absence of pigment
   B. remnants of the hyaloid artery
   C. retinal hemorrhages
   D. clear disc margins
   E. multiple areas of detachment

964. Hyperopia is characterized by all of the following EXCEPT
   A. hyperopic eye is shorter than normal
   B. focused image falls posterior to retina
   C. hyperopia of more than four diopters is considered abnormal in children
   D. in hyperopia of less than four diopters active therapy is needed
   E. proper lenses may correct the condition

965. Dyslexia is a result of
   A. astigmatism
   B. strabismus
   C. myopia
   D. hyperopia
   E. none of the above

966. Astigmatism in a child is usually associated with all of the following EXCEPT
   A. a difference in the refractive power of various corneal meridians, owing to irregularity in the shape of the eyeball
   B. symptoms may include headache, eye pain, fatigue, and conjunctival injection
   C. it may be combined with myopia
   D. it may be combined with hyperopia
   E. all cases of astigmatism require continual use of prescriptive eyeglasses

967. Which of the following is often associated with seborrhea?
   A. Hordeolum
   B. Acute chalazion
   C. Blepharitis
   D. Ectropion
   E. Acute uveitis

968. A three-day-old baby is found to have an acute onset of copious, purulent eye discharge. The conjunctiva are markedly erythematous and the lids are swollen. The most likely diagnosis and course of action are
   A. acute conjunctivitis; treat with saline eye drops
   B. inclusion blennorrhea conjunctivitis; treat with sulfonamide
   C. epidemic keratoconjunctivitis; do not treat
   D. trauma; patch the eyes
   E. no diagnosis until results of smears and cultures are available

969. Epidemic keratoconjunctivitis is characterized by
   A. adenovirus type 8, which can be transmitted by direct contact
   B. ulcerations of the cornea
   C. lack of systemic symptoms
   D. lack of difficulties with visual acuity
   E. a high incidence of blindness

970. Symblepharon is
   A. a perforation from the anterior chamber to the posterior chamber
   B. a detachment of the iris
   C. a coloboma that involves the iris, eyelid, and cornea
   D. a cicatricial attachment of conjunctiva of the lid to the eyeball
   E. an acute conjunctivitis caused by Koch-Weeks bacilli

971. In Holmes-Adie syndrome
   A. one pupil is myotonic and is larger than its counterpart
   B. bilateral cataracts cause blindness
   C. the anterior chamber of the eye fills with blood
   D. the retina swells and overlaps the optic nerve
   E. the eyelid twitches involuntarily

972. Dislocation of the lens has been associated with all of the following EXCEPT
   A. Marchesani syndrome
   B. arachnodactyly
   C. homocystinuria
   D. maternal rubella
   E. trauma

973. All of the following are characteristic of Horner's syndrome EXCEPT
    A. it is a disturbance of cervical sympathetic chain
    B. enophthalmos is apparent
    C. an absence of facial sweating
    D. unilateral miosis
    E. cocaine causes dilation of pupil

974. The earliest and most common finding associated with infantile congenital glaucoma is
    A. tearing
    B. photophobia
    C. strabismus
    D. cupping of the optic disk
    E. megalocornea

975. Strabismus often results in
    A. amblyopia ex anopsia
    B. photophobia
    C. chorioretinitis
    D. infantile glaucoma
    E. conjunctivitis

976. Amblyopia ex anopsia is best treated at
    A. six years
    B. eight years
    C. ten years
    D. 12 years
    E. an early age, before six years

977. The early symptoms of iritis include
    A. diplopia, cataract, and strabismus
    B. conjunctivitis, lid edema, and "ring around the eye"
    C. exophthalmos, headache, and nasal drainage
    D. corneal clouding, itching, and strabismus
    E. none of the above

978. Posterior uveitis can be caused by all of the following EXCEPT
- **A.** toxoplasmosis
- **B.** tuberculosis
- **C.** syphilis
- **D.** vitamin C deficiency
- **E.** brucellosis

979. Chorioretinitis is associated with all of the following EXCEPT
- **A.** syphilis
- **B.** tuberculosis
- **C.** cytomegalic inclusion disease
- **D.** blepharitis
- **E.** visual losses

980. Retinoblastoma is associated with all of the following EXCEPT
- **A.** it is a malignant retinal tumor
- **B.** it usually occurs before age five years
- **C.** it is characterized by the early sign of unilateral nystagmus or strabismus
- **D.** it rarely metastasizes
- **E.** reported familial inheritance

981. A child presents with a cherry red spot in the macula, optic atrophy, progressive ophthalmoplegia, and finally blindness. The most likely diagnosis is
- **A.** Alport's syndrome
- **B.** Tay-Sachs disease
- **C.** aniridia
- **D.** Sieman syndrome
- **E.** Bonnevie-Ullrich syndrome

982. All of the following are associated with optic atrophy EXCEPT
- **A.** Pelizaeus-Merzbacher disease (diffuse cerebral sclerosis)
- **B.** Charcot-Marie-Tooth disease
- **C.** cri-du-chat syndrome
- **D.** Krabbe's syndrome (globoid cell sclerosis)
- **E.** polyostotic fibrous dysplasia

983. The most common ocular complications of diabetes mellitus are found in the
    A. iris
    B. lens
    C. fundus
    D. optic nerve
    E. extraocular muscles

984. The most common primary malignant orbital tumor in children is
    A. rhabdomyosarcoma
    B. glioma of the optic nerve
    C. meningioma
    D. carcinoma
    E. dermoid cyst

DIRECTIONS: Each set of lettered headings below is followed by a list of numbered words or phrases. For each numbered word or phrase select

    A if the item is associated with (A) *only,*
    B if the item is associated with (B) *only,*
    C if the item is associated with *both* (A) *and* (B),
    D if the item is associated with *neither* (A) *nor* (B).

    A. Hyperopia
    B. Myopia
    C. Both
    D. Neither

985. Eyeball is longer than normal, and the focused image falls anterior to the retina

986. Eyeball is shorter than normal, and the focused image falls posterior to the retina

987. A hereditary tendency is found

988. If suspected, total refracture error for full correction should be determined and proper lenses should be worn

989. May be found combined with astigmatism

Directions Summarized			
A	B	C	D
only	only	only	neither
A	B	A,B	A nor B

    A. Gonococcal ophthalmia neonatorum
    B. Inclusion blenorrhea
    C. Both
    D. Neither

990. Prevented by silver nitrate prophylaxis

991. Associated with acute redness and swelling of the lids and profuse exudate

992. Systemic antibiotics are indicated

993. High morbidity even with adequate therapy

994. Causative organism is acquired from the genital tract

    A. Cataract
    B. Uveitis
    C. Both
    D. Neither

995. May be caused by *Toxocara canis*

996. Seen in patients with galactosemia

997. After trauma to one eye, it may appear in the previously unaffected eye

998. Frequently seen in congenital rubella infection

999. Can be a cause of blindness

XIX: Eye
Answers and Comments

950. A. Although a precise determination of visual acuity can be made in a child three to four years of age, with the use of a Snellen "E" chart, visual acuity can be assessed in an infant age six to eight weeks. At this age, the infant should be able to follow a light (or large object) held close to the face. The range may be short, but failure to follow may indicate decreased visual acuity. *(REF. 1 — p. 1943)*

951. D. At birth the eye is 75% that of the adult size; adult size is reached by approximately age eight years. *(REF. 1 — p. 1943)*

952. E. The child at age four to five years has a visual acuity level like that of an adult (20/20). At birth the visual acuity is approximately 20/400. By age three to four years the child can be tested using the Snellen "E" chart. *(REF. 1 — p. 1943)*

953. D. Color vision deficiency is a sex-linked recessive disorder. It occurs in 7.5% of white males, 4.0% of black males but only in 0.6% of all girls. *(REF. 1 — p. 1943)*

954. A. Leukokoria ("white pupillary reflex") is caused by several intraocular diseases but is most often seen with cataract, retinoblastoma, nematode endophthalmitis, and retrolental fibroplasia. *(REF. 1 — p. 1944)*

955. C. Coloboma is usually bilateral and is located inferiorly. The defect usually involves the iris and produces a characteristic "keyhole" defect. *(REF. 1 — p. 1945)*

956. B. Drooping of the upper lid is usually unilateral but not uncommonly it is bilateral, and is secondary to defective development, or absence, of the muscle of the eyelid (the levator muscle). The deficit may be inherited as an autosomal dominant trait. *(REF. 1 — p. 1946)*

957. A. The Marcus Gunn phenomenon results from an anomalous connection between the external pterygoid muscle and the levator muscle. *(REF. 1 — p. 1946)*

958. B. External hordeolum is a pyogenic infection of the ciliary follicle and associated sebaceous glands along the lid margin. Infection is usually caused by staphylococcus. *(REF. 1 — p. 1946)*

959. B. The clinical description and microscopic findings are most compatible with angular blepharitis caused by *H. duplex;* a type of squamous blepharitis, the organism described is also called the diplobacillus of Morax-Axenfeld. *(REF. 1 — p. 1946)*

960. E. The inflammation is sterile. Usually no specific treatment is necessary. On occasion antibiotics are used when there is secondary infection. Permanent damage is rare. *(REF. 1 — p. 1947)*

961. C. The offending organism in trachoma is a virus that belongs to the psittacosis-lymphogranuloma venereum group: chlamydia. Corticosteroids reactivate this virus and are contraindicated. *(REF. 1 — pp. 1948-1949)*

962. E. There is nothing pathognomonic of blueness of the sclera. It can only be said to indicate thinness of the sclera. *(REF. 2 — p. 1939)*

963. E. Detachments are not seen. All of the other features may be observed in a newborn, particularly a premature newborn. The retinal hemorrhages absorb spontaneously and usually have no sequelae. *(REF. 2 — p. 1939)*

964. D. In hyperopia of less than four diopters, it is probable that the power of accommodation is sufficient to supplement the refracting power. Constant use may result in fatigue and ocular discomfort. *(REF. 2 — p. 1942)*

965. E. Dyslexia is a reading disability in which the peripheral organ (the eye) is intact, but the nervous system is deficient in interpreting or making symbolic sense of symbols such as letters and words. *(REF. 2 — p. 1958)*

966. E. Slight astigmatism requires no corrective eyeglasses. Moderate degrees may require the use of lenses for reading, watching TV or movies, or close work. Severe degrees will require continual use of eyeglasses. *(REF. 2 — p. 1943)*

967. C. Blepharitis is an inflammation involving the margins of the eyelids and skin around the cilia. Common findings are erythema, scales, crusts, and ulcerations. Lashes are often matted by debris and exudate. Seborrhea, with or without secondary infection, is a common cause. *(REF. 2 — p. 1965)*

968. E. None of the diagnoses or therapies is acceptable. The history does not rule out gonorrheal conjunctivitis. The proper course is to prepare smears and cultures. If positive for gonorrheal infection, therapy should be instituted with systemic penicillin and local chemotherapy. *(REF. 2 — p. 1967)*

969. A. All of the statements are incorrect except for the etiology and transmission. Corneal changes are rare except for subepithelial corneal infiltrates that can cause blurring of vision. At least 50% of children have systemic symptoms such as fever, sore throat, and malaise. *(REF. 2 — p. 1968)*

970. D. The lower lid is usually involved in the cicatricial attachment to the eyeball. It may be seen following injuries (especially burns) and operations. When it interferes with movement of the eyeball it can cause diplopia. *(REF. 2 — p. 1969)*

971. A. An absence of the Achilles and patellar reflexes is often associated with this pupil abnormality. There is a slow contraction of the pupil in response to direct light, and it remains contracted for a long time. The normal pupil fails to respond to 2.5% methacholine, but the involved pupil responds. *(REF. 2 — p. 1794)*

972. D. Maternal rubella is not usually associated with dislocation of the lens; it is associated with congenital cataract. *(REF. 2 — p. 1970)*

973. E. The reverse is true: pupils fail to dilate with cocaine. However, the pupils dilate with epinephrine, 1:1,000. The normal pupil does not respond to epinephrine. *(REF. 2 — p. 1960)*

974. A. Tearing is the most common sign. The increased intraocular pressure may be present at birth or become apparent in the first three years of life. The tearing must be differentiated from congenital obstruction of the nasolacrimal duct. *(REF. 2 — p. 1977)*

975. A. The major complication of an imbalance of the extraocular muscles is the functional loss of vision, amblyopia ex anopsia. The term implies poor vision resulting from disuse and absence of fusion. *(REF. 2 — p. 1943)*

976. E. Amblyopia ex anopsia is treated at as early an age as possible. Therapy must begin before age six years in order to save vision. Salvage rate is only 40% in the age group four to seven years but is 80% in the age group two to four years. *(REF. 2 — p. 1957)*

977. E. The characteristic early signs of iritis are pain, photophobia, and lacrimation. *(REF. 2 — p. 1970)*

978. D. In addition, posterior uveitis may be found in association with brucellosis, cytomegalic inclusion disease, and as a complication of septicemia. *(REF. 2 — p. 1971)*

979. D. All of the choices given are associated with chorioretinitis except for blepharitis. The areas of the retina involved are ill-defined and yellowish and progress to organized, atrophic white areas with pigmented margins. Visual losses are related to the areas of the retina involved. *(REF. 2 — p. 1971)*

980. D. Retinoblastoma is highly malignant and metastasizes by direct extension into the optic nerve and brain. The tumor is bilateral in about one third of cases. About 6% are familial (autosomal dominant inheritance). *(REF. 2 — p. 1972)*

981. B. The findings are characteristic of amaurotic familial idiocy (Tay-Sachs disease). The other disorders cited may all be associated with cataracts and other ocular disorders. *(REF. 2 — p. 1973)*

982. C. Cri-du-chat syndrome (deletion of the short arm of chromosome number 5) is usually *not* associated with optic atrophy. The characteristic ocular manifestations in this syndrome are hypertelorism, epicanthus, and strabismus. *(REF. 2 — pp. 1945–1946, 1976)*

983. C. The earliest changes in the retina include punctate hemorrhages and microaneurysms. Later in the disease the veins are dilated and tortuous. Small, waxy, yellow exudates appear in the macular area and later over the posterior portion. Scar tissue results in visual loss. *(REF. 2 — p. 1975)*

984. A. The dermoid cyst is common but it is a benign tumor. Of the malignant variety, the rhabdomyosarcoma is the most common. *(REF. 2 — p. 1978)*

985. B. In myopia the eye is longer than normal, and the focused
986. A. image falls anterior to the retina, whereas in hyperopia the
987. B. eye is shorter than normal, and the focused image falls
988. C. posterior to the retina. A hereditary tendency is found in
989. C. myopia, and the children of myopic parents should be ex-
amined. Patients with hyperopia and myopia should have
refractive error determined and wear corrective lenses. Both hyperopia and myopia may also be found in combination with astigmatism. *(REF. 2 — pp. 1942-1943)*

990. A. Both gonococcal ophthalmia and inclusion blenorrhea are
991. C. associated with acute redness and swelling of the lids and
992. A. the production of exudate and both are acquired from the
993. D. genital tract. Neither is associated with great morbidity
994. C. after adequate therapy. In gonococcal ophthalmia systemic
antibiotics are indicated, but silver nitrate prophylaxis is
effective; it is not effective for inclusion blenorrhea. *(REF. 1 — p. 1947)*

995. B. Both cataracts and uveitis can be a cause of blindness.
996. A. Cataracts are frequently seen in patients with galac-
997. B. tosemia and in congenital rubella, but uveitis is not. Uveitis
998. A. may be caused by toxacara infection and may be seen in
999. C. the unaffected eye after trauma to the other eye. Cataracts
are not seen in these circumstances. *(REF. 1 — p. 1957, 1959)*

XX: Ear, Nose, and Throat

DIRECTIONS: Each of the questions or incomplete statements below is followed by five suggested answers or completions. Select the **one** that is **BEST** in each case.

1000. Kartagener's syndrome is characterized by all of the following EXCEPT
    A. situs inversus
    B. bronchiectasis
    C. chronic sinusitis
    D. choanal atresia
    E. aplasia of frontal sinuses

1001. The LEAST common bacterial organism associated with acute sinusitis is
    A. pneumococcus
    B. *S. aureus*
    C. beta-hemolytic streptococcus
    D. *H. influenzae*
    E. *E. coli*

1002. The most common malignant tumor observed in the nose and paranasal sinuses of children is
    A. rhabdomyosarcoma
    B. olfactory epithelioma
    C. lymphoma
    D. renal metastatic tumor
    E. angiofibromas

1003. The most common benign pharyngeal tumor of childhood is
    A. lymphangioma
    B. dermoid
    C. juvenile angiofibroma
    D. neurofibroma
    E. teratoma

1004. Waardenburg syndrome is associated with all of the following EXCEPT
    A. congenital deafness
    B. heterochromia of iris
    C. narrow nasal bridge
    D. white forelock
    E. autosomal-dominant inheritance

1005. Pendred's syndrome is associated with all of the following EXCEPT
    A. congenital deafness
    B. autosomal-recessive inheritance
    C. goiter
    D. retinitis pigmentosa
    E. thyroid abnormality due to inability to change inorganic to organic iodine

1006. Which of the following does NOT characterize Treacher Collins' syndrome?
    A. Autosomal dominant with variable penetrance
    B. Antimongoloid slanting of the eyes
    C. Neurosensory hearing loss
    D. Hypoplasia of facial bone
    E. Coloboma

1007. The most common causative agent associated with external otitis is
    A. *S. aureus*
    B. beta-hemolytic streptococcus
    C. *Pseudomonas aeruginosa*
    D. pneumococcus
    E. *E. coli*

1008. Which of the following does NOT characterize Alport's syndrome?
   A. Autosomal dominance with variable penetrance
   B. Progressive high-tone hearing loss
   C. Glomerulonephritis
   D. Renal tubular acidosis
   E. Variable age of onset and rate of progression

1009. Ramsey Hunt's syndrome is associated with all of the following EXCEPT
   A. herpes zoster
   B. neurosensory deafness
   C. facial paralysis
   D. bullous myringitis
   E. involvement of external auditory canal

XX: Ear, Nose, and Throat
Answers and Comments

1000. D. Choanal atresia is the most common congenital malformation of the nose but is not part of Kartagener's syndrome. *(REF. 1 — p. 948)*

1001. E. *E. coli* is least commonly seen in acute bacterial ingestion of the paranasal sinuses. *(REF. 1 — p. 949)*

1002. A. Malignant tumors are rare in the nose and parasinuses in children, but when present the most common is the rhabdomyosarcoma. *(REF. 1 — p. 949)*

1003. C. Juvenile angiofibromas usually occur in boys and are first noticed at five to six years of age. They are the most common benign tumors in this area. *(REF. 1 — p. 956)*

1004. C. There is lateral displacement of the inner canthi of the eyes and a prominent broad nasal root. *(REF. 1 — p. 967)*

1005. D. Retinitis pigmentosa associated with deafness is known as Usher's syndrome. *(REF. 1 — p. 967)*

1006. C. Hearing loss is usually conductive because of the malformation of the external auditory canal and middle ear. *(REF. 1 — p. 968)*

1007. C. Pseudomonal infections are associated with marked edema of the auditory canal and extreme pain exacerbated by movement of the pinna. *(REF. 1 — p. 968)*

1008. D. Renal tubular acidosis with neurosensory hearing loss may be seen in autosomal recessive disease. *(REF. 1 — p. 970)*

1009. D. The tympanic membrane is usually not involved in this viral infection. *(REF. 1 — p. 972)*

XXI: Skin

DIRECTIONS: Each of the questions or incomplete statements below is followed by five suggested answers or completions. Select the **one** that is **BEST** in each case.

1010. Granuloma annulare is characterized by all of the following EXCEPT
   A. in children it usually disappears spontaneously
   B. usually occurs on trunk
   C. tends to be asymptomatic
   D. unknown etiology
   E. possible peripheral extension of papules or nodules

1011. The characteristics of dermatitis herpetiformis include all of the following EXCEPT
   A. occurrence in generally healthy children
   B. blood eosinophilia is common
   C. it is caused by herpesvirus
   D. the grouped, symmetrical vesicles, or bullae, frequently exacerbate and go into remission spontaneously
   E. urticarial lesions may predominate in mild cases

1012. Toxic epidermal necrolysis (scalded skin syndrome, Lyell's disease) is associated with all of the following EXCEPT
   A. it is most common in infants and young children
   B. group A beta-hemolytic streptococcus is the etiologic agent
   C. the entire skin including palms and soles may be involved as well mucous membranes
   D. in children the clinical course is characterized by spontaneous improvement
   E. Nikolsky's sign is usually positive

1013. Erythema multiforme is characteristically associated with all of the following EXCEPT
   A. relatively asymptomatic skin lesions
   B. with involvement of conjunctivitis and mucous membranes the disease is sometimes called Stevens-Johnson syndrome
   C. lesions include macules, purpuric spots, urticaria, vesicles and bullae
   D. the cause is unknown in most cases
   E. polymorphonuclear leukocytes usually predominate in the vesicular fluid

1014. Cellulitis occurring about the face in young children (six to 24 months) and associated with fever and a purple skin discoloration is most often caused by
   A. group A beta-hemolytic streptococci
   B. *H. influenzae*
   C. *S. pneumococci*
   D. *S. aureus*
   E. pseudomonas

1015. Erythrasma is associated with all of the following EXCEPT
   A. asymptomatic disease with cutaneous appearance in toe webs, axilla, and inguinal regions
   B. it is caused by fungal organisms
   C. coral-red fluorescence is noted on Wood's light examination
   D. topical salicylic acid ointment is the treatment of choice
   E. it is commonly confused with tinea pedis

1016. Which of the following is FALSE regarding varicella-viral infections?
   A. Man is the only natural host
   B. Chickenpox is a result of exposure to the virus of a susceptible individual
   C. Zoster is thought to be caused by reactivation of latent varicella virus
   D. Zoster may affect any area of the body
   E. Zoster is not contagious

1017. Herpes zoster is associated with all of the following EXCEPT
  A. demonstration of intracytoplasmic inclusions by biopsy of lesions
  B. antibody may be found in both "slow" and "fast" IgG components
  C. persistent or severe pain during active disease is unusual in children, and postherpetic neuralgia is rare in childhood
  D. lesions characterized by grouped vesicles are located in the distribution of the infected spinal or cranial sensory nerves
  E. Guillain-Barré syndrome

1018. Molluscum contagiosum is characterized by all of the following EXCEPT
  A. its only natural host is man
  B. unknown etiology
  C. lesions are discrete, nearly gray umbilicated papules
  D. autoinoculation is common
  E. may appear at any age

1019. The description, asymptomatic, superficial, confluent, non-erythematous, scaly dermatitis that does not fluoresce, best fits infection with which of the following fungal organisms?
  A. *Malassezia furfur*
  B. *Microsporum canis*
  C. *M. audouinii*
  D. *Trichophyton tonsurans*
  E. *Epidermophyton floccosum*

1020. Tinea capitus is associated with all of the following EXCEPT
  A. it is most often due to infection with microsporum species
  B. the lesions frequently fluoresce with Wood's lamp examination
  C. it is occasionally associated with kerion
  D. may be transmitted from animals to man
  E. easily treated with local fungistatic preparations

1021. Incontinentia pigmenti is characterized by all of the following EXCEPT
   A. it occurs almost exclusively in males
   B. irregular whorled patterns of pigmentation
   C. dental abnormalities
   D. disorders of central nervous system
   E. first signs of the disease are linear or grouped vesicles

1022. Pityriasis rosea is characterized by all of the following EXCEPT
   A. it is a papulosquamous disease primarily of the trunk
   B. herald patch
   C. pruritus is most common symptom
   D. prodrome of cough, fever, and conjunctivitis
   E. color, distribution, and morphology of the lesions are usually sufficient to establish a diagnosis.

DIRECTIONS: For each of the questions or incomplete statements below, **ONE** or **MORE** of the answers or completions given is correct. Select
   A if only *1, 2 and 3* are correct,
   B if only *1 and 3* are correct,
   C if only *2 and 4* are correct,
   D if only *4* is correct,
   E if all are correct.

1023. The compartments of the epidermis include
   1. stratum corneum
   2. malpighian, or prickle-cell, layer
   3. basal, or "stem cell," layer
   4. stratum epithelium

1024. In nonbullous congenital ichthyosiform erythroderma (CIE)
   1. mental retardation and spastic paralysis may occur
   2. an autosomal recessive mode of transmission is observed
   3. ectropion is common
   4. the harlequin fetus appearance may be present

Directions Summarized				
A	B	C	D	E
1,2,3	1,3	2,4	4	All are
only	only	only	only	correct

1025. Patients with herpes zoster
    1. benefit from definitive therapy
    2. may have involvement of the cornea
    3. suffer little discomfort even in the face of widespread disease
    4. are contagious

1026. In the approach to the patient with pyoderma
    1. the infection should be considered to be mixed, with both strep and staph present
    2. septicemia should be considered a common problem
    3. systemic antibiotics are considered to be superior to local therapy
    4. family screening for carriers is not necessary

1027. Toxic epidermal necrolysis (TEN) may be associated with
    1. staphylococcal infection
    2. streptococcal infection
    3. desquamation
    4. very high mortality in infants

1028. Erythema multiforme has been associated with
    1. streptococcal infections
    2. drug sensitization
    3. connective tissue diseases
    4. tuberculosis

1029. Vascular nevi that require no treatment and usually resolve spontaneously include
    1. cavernous hemangioma
    2. nevus flammeus
    3. nevus araneus
    4. strawberry hemangioma

1030. The history, symptoms, and signs of pityriasis rosea may include
    1. infrequent onset of febrile illness as a prodrome
    2. presence of pruritus
    3. papulosquamous rash that may be vesicular
    4. scarring, which is frequently seen

1031. Patients with eczema have been shown to have
    1. family history of atopy
    2. hyperactive T cells
    3. abnormal response to intracutaneous methacholine
    4. abnormal macrophage inhibitory factor (MIF) response

1032. Conditions associated with hypopigmentation include
    1. Waardenburg's syndrome
    2. Mucha-Habermann disease
    3. Chédiak-Steinbrinck-Higashi syndrome
    4. ephelides

XXI: Skin
Answers and Comments

1010. B. Characteristically, the back of hands and fingers and extensor aspects of the arms and legs are involved. *(REF. 1 — p. 865)*

1011. C. The etiology is unknown, although it is thought not to be an infectious process. *(REF. 1 — p. 871)*

1012. B. Lyell's disease is most often associated with a toxin from the coagulase-positive phage group 2 staphylococci. *(REF. 1 — p. 873)*

1013. E. Eosinophils may be present, but lymphocytes usually predominate. *(REF. 1 — p. 874)*

1014. B. Cellulitis caused by staphylococcal and streptococcal disease is usually associated with pyoderma (papulovesicular lesions). Pneumococcal infections are rarely associated with cellulitis. Pseudomonal infections associated with septicemia may be seen in ulcerative lesions. *(REF. 1 — p. 878)*

1015. B. Erythrasma is caused by a gram-positive bacillus, corynebacterium. *(REF. 1 — p. 878)*

1016. E. Zoster is contagious for at least five to seven days after vesicles appear in affected patients. *(REF. 1 — p. 879)*

1017. A. Inclusion bodies are intranuclear in zoster but are intracytoplasmic in smallpox. *(REF. 1 — p. 880)*

1018. B. Molluscum is classified as a poxvirus. *(REF. 1 — p. 880)*

1019. A. The description is characteristic of tinea versicolor. *(REF. 1 — p. 883)*

1020. E. Infection of the hair and hair shafts usually requires systemic administration of griseofulvin. *(REF. 1 — p. 884)*

1021. A. Occurs almost exclusively in infant females. *(REF. 1 — p. 897)*

1022. D. Prodrome is rare but may be infrequently associated with low grade fever and sore throat. *(REF. 1 — p. 902)*

1023. A. The layers of the epidermis are the basal cell layer, the prickle, or malpighian, layer, and the stratum corneum. *(REF. 1 — p. 853)*

1024. E. Nonbullous CIE is characterized by autosomal recessive mode of inheritance and generalized ichthyosis. Ectropion is common. In its severe form, harlequin fetus appears. When associated with mental retardation and spasticity the term Sjögren-Larsson syndrome is used. *(REF. 1 — p. 856)*

1025. C. Herpes zoster is contagious in affected patients for five to seven days after vesicles appear and corneal involvement may be present. There is no definitive therapy, and pain is the rule rather than the exception, even with minor involvement. *(REF. 1 — p. 878)*

1026. B. Pyoderma is usually a mixed infection of both staph and strep. Systemic antibiotics are far superior to local therapy. Family contact should be screened to detect carriers. Sepsis is an uncommon complication of pyoderma. *(REF. 1 — p. 877)*

1027. B. TEN is associated with staphylococcal (phage group 2) infection and widespread desquamation. Death is uncommon in infants. *(REF. 1 — p. 872)*

1028. E. All of the conditions listed have been associated with erythema multiforme as have mycoplasma, herpes simplex, and deep mycoses. *(REF. 1 — p. 874)*

1029. D. Cavernous hemangioma and nevus flammeus (port wine stain) do not resolve spontaneously. *(REF. 1 — p. 905)*

1030. A. Pityriasis rosea infrequently is preceded by a febrile illness as a prodrome and never produces scarring without 2° infection. The rash, which is papulosquamous and may be vesicular, is frequently pruritic. *(REF. 1 — pp. 902–903)*

1031. B. Patients with eczema have been shown to have a high incidence of family history of atopy and an abnormal methacholine test as evidenced by delayed blanching. They do not have hyperactive neutrophils or abnormal MIF response. *(REF. 1 — p. 899)*

1032. B. Waardenburg's and Chédiak-Steinbrinck-Higashi syndromes are associated with patterned leukoderma and albinism, respectively. Mucha-Habermann disease and ephelides (freckles) are not associated with hypopigmentation. *(REF. 1 — p. 895)*

XXII: Teeth

Each of the questions or incomplete statements below is followed by five suggested answers or completions. Select the **one** that is **BEST** in each case.

1033. When does the dental lamina initiate development of the permanent teeth?
   A. Fourth to fifth month in utero
   B. Ninth month in utero
   C. One year postnatally
   D. Two years postnatally
   E. Three years postnatally

1034. Calcification of the primary teeth occurs
   A. in the first six months of life
   B. in the second six months of life
   C. both prenatally and postnatally
   D. entirely in utero and is complete at 36 weeks gestation
   E. only after eruption begins

1035. In regard to the eruption of teeth, which of the following situations is ABNORMAL?
   A. First tooth at four months
   B. First tooth at six months
   C. First tooth at eight months
   D. Permanent central incisor at seven months
   E. First tooth at 16 months

1036. All of the following might be possible etiologies for discoloration of the teeth of a 15-month-old infant EXCEPT

    A. iron medication

    B. dental decay

    C. tetracycline given to mother during pregnancy

    D. breast-feeding

    E. improper fluoride administration

1037. Nighttime bottle caries can be prevented by

    A. toothbrushing in the morning

    B. the substitution of juice for milk

    C. only using milk in bottle

    D. using only sugar water at naptime

    E. not giving a bottle at naptime or bedtime

1038. Fluoridation of the water supply has been associated with

    A. a reduction in decay of more than 60%

    B. overall support of the practice by the dental and medical profession

    C. increased incidence of early dental eruption

    D. increased incidence of delayed dental eruption

    E. no appreciable reduction in decay

XXII: Teeth
Answers and Comments

1033. A. The permanent central incisors development first begins at about the fifth month in utero. Development of the other permanent teeth continues at various times until about ten months postnatally. *(REF. 1 — pp. 932–933)*

1034. C. Calcification of the primary teeth begins at about four months in utero and is complete at ten to 12 months postnatally. *(REF. 1 — p. 933)*

1035. E. Infrequently the first tooth will not erupt until 12 months of age. Eruption occurring later than this would require investigation. *(REF. 1 — pp. 934–935)*

1036. D. Other causes of dental discoloration include trauma, and tetracycline administration during infancy. *(REF. 1 — pp. 936–941)*

1037. E. Any sugar-containing fluid nursed by the infant at naptime or nighttime is a potential caries producer. The upper teeth usually show signs of disease before the lower teeth. *(REF. 1 — pp. 941–942)*

1038. A. While not all professional health groups are convinced of the safety and effectiveness of fluoridation, studies demonstrate significant reduction in dental decay. *(REF. 1 — p. 941)*

XXIII: Unclassified Disorders

DIRECTIONS: Each of the questions or incomplete statements below is followed by five suggested answers or completions. Select the **one** that is **BEST** in each case.

1039. The incidence of crib death in rural areas of the United States is
   A. higher than the urban rate
   B. equal to death rates in the city
   C. approximately 1.2/1000 live births
   D. the same as that reported in Ireland and East Germany
   E. none of the above

1040. In sudden infant death syndrome, an identifiable cause of death at autopsy will be found in what percentage of cases?
   A. 50%
   B. 1%
   C. 5%
   D. 25%
   E. 15%

1041. The peak incidence of crib death occurs at
   A. five to six months
   B. one to two months
   C. two to four months
   D. six to eight months
   E. two to four weeks

1042. Which of the following statements is true concerning crib death?
  A. Females are more commonly involved
  B. Prematures are rarely involved
  C. Increased incidence in summer in Northeastern states
  D. Never reported in breast-fed infants
  E. None of the above

1043. Which of the following is true of most crib deaths?
  A. They occur between 1 PM and 4 PM
  B. They occur between 8 PM and 12 AM
  C. They occur between 12 AM and 9 AM
  D. They occur between 8 AM and 12 PM
  E. There is no relationship to time of day

1044. Which of the following factors is NOT associated with increased risk of sudden infant death syndrome?
  A. Lower socioeconomic status
  B. Illegitimate birth
  C. Young mother with high parity
  D. Infant age of two to four months
  E. Spotting during first trimester

1045. The death rate for siblings of crib death infants from the same cause is in what relationship to that of the population at large?
  A. The same
  B. Four to seven times greater
  C. Less
  D. 20 times greater
  E. 50 times greater

1046. The cause of sudden infant death is
  A. pulmonary hemorrhage
  B. suffocation
  C. CNS hemorrhage
  D. pulmonary aspiration of vomitus
  E. unknown

1047. The number of crib deaths that occur annually in the U.S. is estimated to be at least
  A. 2,000
  B. 30,000
  C. 6,000-7,000
  D. 20,000
  E. 50,000

1048. Patients with familial Mediterranean fever display all of the following EXCEPT
  A. a positive rectal biopsy for amyloid
  B. renal failure
  C. autosomal recessive inheritance
  D. occurrence primarily among ethnic groups originating from the Mediterranean area
  E. amyloidosis, which is felt to be a secondary phenomenon

1049. Children with sarcoidosis are more likely to be
  A. caucasian
  B. urban
  C. more than ten years of age
  D. afebrile
  E. asymptomatic

1050. The organ most frequently affected in sarcoidosis is
  A. kidney
  B. lung
  C. heart
  D. brain
  E. spleen

1051. Which of the following is (are) useful in the treatment of sarcoidosis?
  A. Megavitamins
  B. Corticosteroids
  C. Streptomycin
  D. Antituberculosis drugs and corticosteroids
  E. Calcium

1052. Which of the following is known to be associated with the histocytosis syndromes?
   A. Occurrence in males is more common
   B. Malignancy
   C. Transmissable to animals
   D. Familial origin
   E. Occurrence in females is more common

1053. What percentage of patients with histiocytosis present with bone lesions only?
   A. 50%
   B. 25%
   C. 75%
   D. 10%
   E. 5%

1054. In which year of life does the patient with Letterer-Siwe disease usually present with symptoms?
   A. Twelfth
   B. Seventh
   C. Third
   D. Fifth
   E. First

1055. The clinical type of histiocytosis with the highest mortality is
   A. Letterer-Siwe disease
   B. Hand-Schüller-Christian disease
   C. eosinophilic granuloma
   D. sarcoidosis
   E. none of the above are associated with mortality

1056. Patients with histiocytosis classified as Hand-Schüller-Christian disease usually present at
   A. eight to ten years
   B. three to five years
   C. 12 to 15 years
   D. ten to 12 years
   E. two to three years

1057. Which of the following is LEAST likely to alleviate symptoms when used in the management of the histiocytosis syndrome?
    A. Radiotherapy
    B. Corticosteroids
    C. Alkylating agents
    D. Folic acid antagonists
    E. Antibacterial drugs

1058. Features of progeria include all of the following EXCEPT
    A. short stature
    B. sexual infantilism
    C. little subcutaneous fat
    D. hirsutism
    E. aged appearance of facial features

1059. The Wechsler Intelligence Scale for Children — Revised (WISC-R) is characterized by all of the following EXCEPT
    A. useful in age range two years to ten years
    B. provides a verbal IQ
    C. provides a full scale IQ
    D. allows for observations of behavior
    E. test results may point to specific areas of dysfunction

1060. Which one of the following is useful in evaluating various aspects of personality, adjustment and self-concept?
    A. WISC-R
    B. McCarthy Scales of Children's Abilities
    C. Stanford-Binet
    D. Wechsler Preschool and Primary Scale of Infant Intelligence
    E. Thematic Apperception Test (TAT)

XXIII: Unclassified Disorders
Answers and Comments

1039. C. The urban rate is approximately 3.1 per 1,000 live births in a typical large city. *(REF. 2 — p. 1647)*

1040. E. At autopsy, approximately 15% of cases of suspected crib deaths will have a definable cause of death. *(REF. 2 — pp. 1980–1981)*

1041. C. Few deaths are attributed to crib death after age six months. *(REF. 2 — p. 1980)*

1042. E. Males and prematures are at increased risk. If there are large temperature changes in a climate, far more deaths occur in the winter. Formula-fed babies have a higher incidence of SIDS than breast-fed infants. *(REF. 2 — p. 1980)*

1043. C. Most deaths occur between 12 AM and 9 AM, suggesting disturbance of sleep as a factor. *(REF. 2 — p. 1980)*

1044. E. The syndrome occurs regardless of socioeconomic status, illegitimacy or high parity in the mother. However, all of these factors significantly increase the risk, and males are more affected than females. The relationship to "spotting" during the first trimester has not been reported. *(REF. 2 — p. 1980)*

1045. B. There is as yet no coherent Mendelian interpretation of this observation. *(REF. 2 — p. 1980)*

1046. E. This type of death probably represents some instantaneous interruption of a control mechanism that results in apnea and bradycardia. *(REF. 2 — p. 1981)*

1047. C. At least 6,000-7,000 infants die annually from SIDS, or crib death. *(REF. 2 — p. 1980)*

1048. E. This disease is classified as a primary amyloidosis because amyloid may be found very early in association with familial Mediteranean fever. *(REF. 2 — p. 1982)*

1049. C. The disease is most common in rural communities and is uncommon in children less than ten years of age. *(REF. 2 — p. 1982)*

1050. B. Parenchymal infiltrates and hilar lymphadenopathy are most often present. *(REF. 2 — p. 1982)*

1051. B. Corticosteroids may be especially helpful in the management of ocular lesions and hypercalcemia. *(REF. 2 — p. 1983)*

1052. A. Males are more common in all clinical groups and younger patients tend to have more disseminated lesions. *(REF. 2 — p. 1984)*

1053. A. One to 12 or more lytic defects may be present; these usually resolve within one to two years. *(REF. 2 — p. 1984)*

1054. E. Most infants are under one year of age. The liver, spleen, marrow, and lungs are involved quite rapidly. *(REF. 2 — pp. 1984–1985)*

1055. A. These patients, because of their deep visceral involvement, have a significant mortality. *(REF. 2 — pp. 1984–1985)*

1056. E. These patients will have osseous lesions and minor additional involvement such as anemia or skin lesions. *(REF. 2 — p. 1984)*

1057. E. Folic acid antagonists have rarely produced favorable results. Antibacterial agents produce no change. *(REF. 2 — p. 1986)*

1058. D. Alopecia is generalized and frequently the skin is dry and wrinkled. *(REF. 2 — pp. 1986–1988)*

1059. A. The age range for the WISC-R is from five years to 15 years 11 months. *(REF. 1 — p. 1787)*

1060. E. Choices A,B,C,D all assess intelligence levels. The TAT is utilized for projective techniques and evaluates the adjustment pattern of the subject. *(REF. 1 — pp. 1787–1789)*

References

1. Rudolph, A.M., Barnett, H.L., and Einhorn, A.H.: *Pediatrics.* 16th Ed. New York: Appleton-Century-Crofts, 1977.
2. Vaughan, V.A. III, McKay, R.J., and Behrman, R.E.: *Nelson Textbook of Pediatrics.* 11th Ed. Philadelphia: W.B. Saunders, 1979.
3. Vaughan, V.A. III, McKay, R.J., and Nelson, W.E.: *Textbook of Pediatrics.* 10th Ed. Philadelphia: W.B. Saunders, 1975.